THE
BODY
LIBERATION
PROJECT

THE
BODY
LIBERATION
PROJECT

HOW UNDERSTANDING RACISM AND
DIET CULTURE HELPS CULTIVATE JOY AND
BUILD COLLECTIVE FREEDOM

Chrissy King

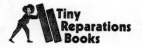
Tiny
Reparations
Books

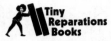

An imprint of Penguin Random House LLC
penguinrandomhouse.com

"Nectar" reprinted with permission from the author.

LIBRARY OF CONGRESS CATALOGING-IN-PUBLICATION DATA
Names: King, Chrissy, author.
Title: The body liberation project: how understanding racism and diet culture helps cultivate joy and build collective freedom / Chrissy King.
Description: New York: Tiny Reparations Books, [2022] |
Includes bibliographical references.
Identifiers: LCCN 2022040224 (print) | LCCN 2022040225 (ebook) |
ISBN 9780593187043 (hardcover) | ISBN 9780593187050 (ebook)
Subjects: LCSH: Body image. | Body image in women. |
African American women. | Self-acceptance. | Racism. |
Social justice. Classification: LCC BF697.5.B63 K569 2022 (print) |
LCC BF697.5.B63 (ebook) | DDC 306.4/613—dc23/eng/20221116
LC record available at https://lccn.loc.gov/2022040224
LC ebook record available at https://lccn.loc.gov/2022040225

Printed in the United States of America
1st Printing

BOOK DESIGN BY ASHLEY TUCKER

THIS BOOK IS DEDICATED TO MY MOM AND DAD. Mom, while I'm almost positive you don't really know what I do for a living or how I pay my bills, I appreciate that your support is relentless. You also personally taught me to read and write, so I guess you can take a lot of the credit for this book. To my dad, although you are no longer here in the physical realm, I'm positive that you're smiling down on me. I know your heart is swelling with pride and you're not the least bit surprised about where life has taken me. I think you saw it all before I did.

Contents

AUTHOR'S NOTE

I wanted to write you a quick note before you jump into reading the book. First of all, I just want to say thank you from the bottom of my heart for taking the time to read my book. Writing a book is a dream come true for me. Younger me, who spent all her time reading books and writing stories, would be so filled with joy to know that one day she would actually write and publish a book. This was a labor of love, filled with so many emotions, but above all, I'm just so grateful that I got this opportunity.

Secondly, I want to tell you that I'm not perfect, nor do I always get it right, despite my best efforts. In writing this book, I did my absolute best to use the most up-to-date terms and to be as inclusive in my language as possible, but as you probably already know, things change frequently. So perhaps by the time you read this, terminology has changed, or maybe I just flat-out got something wrong. I apologize in advance if I've missed the mark on certain topics. I'm continuously learning, growing, and decolonizing my mind. So while I can't promise that I got everything right, I can promise you that I'll never stop striving to get it right.

Finally, I wrote this book through the lens of my own personal experience, and I realize that my experiences can't possibly cover the issues presented from all angles. Despite that, I hope that you feel seen and understood as you read through it, and I invite you to ponder your own personal experiences as you explore the concepts presented.

THE
BODY
LIBERATION
PROJECT

Identity, Representation, and Living in a Marginalized Body

I LOVE BEING BLACK. I LOVE BEING TALL. I LOVE MY BODY. I CELE-brate myself daily. I wrote the ode below to myself some-time last year, and I mean it with every fiber of my being.

> *Sometimes I wonder how I got so lucky.*
> *To be born so Black.*
> *And so woman.*
> *And so magical.*
> *But then I stop questioning it.*
> *Sometimes it just is what it is.*

But if I'm being 100 percent honest, I didn't always feel this way. I definitely didn't grow up celebrating myself. I didn't always bask in my beauty or appreciate the splendor of my being. In fact, my journey of learning to unapologetically love myself has been just that—a journey.

I have early childhood memories of being uncomfortable in my body. I was always a tall child. I was almost five eight by the time I was in the third grade, while most of my peers were averaging four eight—yes, you read that correctly. I was much taller than my mom, and many other adults, at the age of nine. I have a picture from a Thanksgiving celebration at my private middle school that is still etched into my brain. I don't know where the picture is anymore, but that doesn't really matter. I can still see the image vividly. I'm the only Black child in my class, and I'm positioned all the way in the back because I'm taller than everyone, even the teacher. And I'm dressed like a Pilgrim. In hindsight, there were a myriad of issues with this scenario, but give me a break—I was nine. I didn't know about the problematic nature of dressing up as Pilgrims and Native Americans yet. Nonetheless, to say I stuck out like a sore thumb is an understatement.

However, I was never teased by other kids because of my height. My siblings lovingly referred to me as "Jolly Green Giant," but to be honest, that didn't really bother me too much. I never particularly minded being tall, but I was super cognizant of my weight, specifically because of my height. I'm not sure when I adopted this thought process, but in my mind, since I was tall, it was only acceptable that I be thin. If I was destined to be tall, then I should aspire to the slim model look. If I were tall and big, then I would look like a linebacker. I don't remember anyone telling me this. *I just remember thinking this for as long as I can remember.*

Growing up in the Midwest as a Black girl from a working-class family and attending a predominantly affluent, white school made it difficult to truly embrace myself. My hair was thick and coily, while everyone else had long, flowing locks. My family could barely afford the private-school tuition, while my peers were living in fancy, beautifully decorated homes and traveled the world on holidays. Their parents were lawyers and doctors; mine had high school diplomas.

It was the late '90s, and I didn't see myself represented anywhere, especially in fashion magazines and TV ads that promoted messages like "Get flat abs fast" and "Lose 10 pounds in 10 days." You know the ones I'm talking about. They were omnipresent.

Everywhere I turned, there was a standard I couldn't reach.

I couldn't change the color of my skin, nor did I wish to, but I realized *I could* make my body thinner. I could try to be thin and pretty, and I put all my energy into the pursuit. I didn't have the vocabulary or the understanding at that time in my life, but what I was really seeking was access to privilege and proximity to whiteness.

It's funny the memories that never leave you. Around age ten or eleven, I had this deep fuchsia shirt with a half zipper that I absolutely loved—like hands down, my favorite shirt. However, as much as I liked it, something about this shirt made me realize that my stomach poked out. I started walking around my house with my shoulders hunched and slouched to the front with the hope that my family wouldn't notice my gut. In hindsight, I wonder why I didn't just suck my stomach in. Surely, that would have been easier. I secretly hoped no one would notice my "problem area." Then one day, my oldest brother pointed out my attempt to hide my stomach, and I was devastated. I'm sure he doesn't even remember that, *but I never forgot.*

On the other hand, there are certain things that we simply can't remember. I can't remember why, at such a young age, I felt something was wrong with my body. I don't know who I learned these thoughts from. Sometimes I wish I could go back in time and have a conversation with my younger self. Maybe not to tell her that everything will be okay or that my body was fine, but just because I really wish I knew what was going through her head.

I recently found a journal from my childhood dated January 1, 1998. I was twelve years old. Apparently, enough was enough, and I was going to get my body in shape. I wrote:

Today is the day after the church lock in. I got home 6 hours ago. I slept for a while, but I'm still tired. All I've been doing is laying around watching TV. I'm super tired so I don't have much to say. I need to do my exercise for *the day, but I'm too tired. Oh well, I have to do it anyways. Hasta mañana!*

On the previous page of this journal entry, I had written out my diet and exercise plan. I was to exercise at 7 a.m. every day, seven days a week—even when I didn't feel like it. By thirteen, I was keeping a food journal and allowed myself a breakfast of fewer than three hundred calories and three grams of fat. According to another journal entry, I wasn't allowed to eat pizza, chips, or sweets. I also required myself to hop on the scale every day to check my weight. My lunch suggestions included things like a salad with no dressing, a piece of fruit, carrots, twenty-three pretzels (very specific, I know), or one cup of yogurt. For each of the items listed, I included the total number of calories and amount of fat. I believed, as so many of us have been told, that fat was a very bad thing to include in your diet. Last, for dinner, I wrote that I should "try to eat light" and "try to resist dessert." *These were the thoughts on my mind at the tender age of thirteen.*

The interesting thing is that I spent so much time obsessing about being tall and thin, then at some point I grew even taller and in fact became tall and thin. Perhaps it was due to my restrictive diet or simply my growing and changing body. I look back at pictures of myself from the ages of fourteen to sixteen, and I actually looked pretty lanky. I hadn't filled in with many curves yet, although I would soon. But for some reason, even during those lanky years, I saw something different in the reflection in the mirror. Then, at the age of seventeen, I went on my first hard-core diet after a classmate called out my recent weight gain.

I spent nearly the next decade yo-yo dieting. My number one priority was keeping my body in check, at all costs. I couldn't enjoy social events without stressing about food or how my body looked, and I refused to miss a workout, even for something important. I distinctly remember the time I drove to my mom's apartment complex, which had an exercise room, at 11 p.m. to do forty-five minutes of additional cardio because I had eaten a bag of M&M's. I justified these behaviors in the name of being "healthy." But the truth was, *all I really wanted was to shrink my body at whatever cost necessary.*

I JOINED THE GYM FOR THE FIRST TIME IN MY ADULT LIFE AT THE age of twenty-four. I had regained some weight yet again, and I joined the gym with one goal in my mind: get skinny. But if I'm being honest, the real reason I joined the gym is because my baby sister, Celina, had joined the gym and hired a trainer, so I basically was just copying her. Our first trainer was a petite white woman named Megan. During our first official session, Megan discussed that we would be strength training, to which I immediately responded, "I said I want to be skinny, not get muscles." She explained that the way she was going to train me was also how she trained, and because she was skinny, I acquiesced. I hated every moment of my first thirty-minute session with a trainer. But since I had paid for a package of twelve sessions, I kept going. It's important to note that I have since learned that people's bodies are not business cards, and the size and shape of a person's body doesn't predicate their ability to help people reach their personal health and fitness goals. The fact that Megan was petite said zero about her knowledge or skill as a trainer.

Megan also prescribed me a meal plan, at my request. I now also know that it is completely illegal for trainers to give out meal plans unless they are registered dieticians, but I had no idea back then, and my thought process was that if Megan was skinny, then surely she was qualified to help me get skinny as well. That first meal plan she gave me was a thousand-calorie-a-day diet. No adult should be restricting their calorie intake to one thousand calories a day—even toddlers need more calories than that. In Megan's defense, she told me to only follow the diet for thirty days for a "jump start." But when the pounds started melting away and the number on the scale started shrinking, I kept up with the diet for far longer than thirty days. I stayed with Megan way past the initial twelve sessions too, training with her three days a week and adding in copious amounts of cardio. I was literally watching myself shrink before my own eyes. I was thrilled. I later found out that the thousand-calorie-a-day diet was just an exact carbon copy of a diet written by celebrity trainer Jackie Warner from her book *10 Pounds in 10 Days*. Also, as I was writing this, I got curious about what Jackie was up to these days and headed to her Instagram. Turns out she's still promoting that thousand-calorie diet as a way to "jump-start and boost your self-esteem." I guess some things never change.

Then, along the way, an interesting thing happened. I actually started enjoying the process of strength training. I started getting physically stronger, and I liked that feeling. *Perhaps there was more to my body than just what it looked like.* Through a series of events, I found myself training at a small strength and conditioning gym. For the first time in my life, I saw women powerlifting, a strength sport that consists of bench pressing, squatting, and deadlifting with a barbell. I was intrigued, despite the fact that I had never even held a barbell in my hands. After a couple months of casual observation, I was encouraged by the owner to try it for myself, and as cheesy as it sounds, it was love at first lift.

Powerlifting was transformative for me both mentally and physically. I spent the majority of my twenties focused on shrinking—my body, my voice, and my life in general. I was obsessed with my weight and truly believed that my happiness lay on the other side of fat loss. Powerlifting was the first step to changing that mindset. It allowed me to stop focusing all my energy on what my body looked like and to start seeing all that it could do. I finally grasped how strong and capable I was. After a couple of years, I started competing in powerlifting competitions, and eventually was able to regularly deadlift over four hundred pounds. When I was growing up, the running joke was that I was the weakling in the family. No one asked me to do any heavy lifting, and it didn't bother me at all. In my mind, some people were strong and other people were weak; I just happened to be weak. But after falling in love with strength training, I realized that strength is a skill that can be developed just like any other skill. The lessons I learned in the gym also transferred to other areas of my life as well. If the narrative that I was just a weakling wasn't true, what other narratives had I been holding that weren't true? However, despite all these incredible realizations I was having, it wasn't quite enough to end my desire to shrink my body.

Even though I was in the leanest body of my adult life, it was never enough. There were always five more pounds that I needed to lose or a "problem" area that I needed to fix. My sister regularly commented that she thought I was losing my mind because I was so critical of my weight and my body. I'll never forget the meme she jokingly sent me when I was deep in the throes of what should probably be described as body dysmorphia, defined by Mayo Clinic as "a mental health condition in which you can't stop thinking about one or more perceived defects or flaws in your appearance—a flaw that appears minor or can't be seen by others. But you may feel so embarrassed, ashamed and anxious that you may avoid many social situations."

To be clear, this is me diagnosing myself. I never sought

professional help, but I can definitely say that I have never read a more accurate description of my state of mind at that time in my life. The reason that the term "body dysmorphia" resonated with me so deeply is that I was the woman who got constant affirmation from strangers on the street about the appearance of my body. Everyone was constantly validating my appearance, but all I could see were the parts of me that were imperfect. So the part that says "a flaw that appears minor or can't be seen by others" is the definition of how I existed. It didn't matter what anyone else thought or how often I was on the receiving end of compliments about my body and looks, I always felt the same. I still needed "fixing."

Back to the meme. The background was a picture of a skeleton and the caption read, "Bitches be like: 'I finally reached my goal weight.'" My sister sent it as a joke, but there was also a part of her that really believed no matter how much weight I lost, I would never be happy.

Although I never had an eating disorder, there was a time in my life that I feel like I came pretty close. Before working in fitness and becoming a writer, I worked in a professional setting and sat next to a coworker, Ken, who would eventually become one of my best friends. I'm not sure exactly how it started, but he began periodically bringing in donuts from one of my favorite places. I tried to resist most of the time. However, I remember one day I gave in and ended up eating three donuts. I felt so guilty and ashamed, and quite frankly terrified of gaining weight, that I went to the bathroom and made myself throw it all up. This happened three more times on different occasions. I realized how easily I slipped into this pattern, and the thought of developing a full-blown eating disorder scared me enough to stop.

Even though I was the smallest I had been in my adult life, and people constantly complimented my body, I had a horrible body image and an extremely complicated and unhealthy relationship with food, and I was scared of gaining a single pound. I didn't enjoy denying myself the foods I loved, but I had become so indoctrinated in the fitness industry that I wholeheartedly believed the sentiment that "food is fuel." And therefore, pleasure wasn't a part of eating. I prided myself in being disciplined as it pertained to my eating choices, especially my ability to deny myself the right to eat certain foods.

Truth be told, obsessing about food and exercise was really exhausting, and I eventually realized that if I didn't change something, I would always be unhappy with myself, regardless of how thin I got. I started the difficult work of healing my body image. During this journey to heal my relationship with my body (which took several years in total), I gravitated to the online body positivity space—particularly Instagram—and it seemed to me like everyone was having such an easy time accepting their bodies and loving themselves.

Why did I find myself struggling so much?

In my mind, I knew that the system was broken. Wellness was supposed to make me healthier, but I didn't feel well at all. I felt anxious and distracted, and even more, I was miserable. How had deciding to lose weight, and actually accomplishing that goal, led me here?

While having these epiphanies about the way the diet industry intentionally markets to our insecurities, I also began addressing my own issues with body image as a Black woman while navigating an industry that was predominantly white and thin. I began to realize that my inability to feel worthy in my own skin was predicated on so much more than just my individual feelings about my body. As I began to understand the origins of fatphobia and its ties to white supremacy, it became ever more clear to me that my struggles with body image were much bigger than just me.

And to add to that, there were cultural implications. Black girls weren't supposed to struggle with body image, and certainly not eating issues or disorders. No one ever explicitly said that, but young white women were the face of eating disorders, not Black girls. And while Black girls have been left out of the discussion, the reality is that Black women struggle with body image and eating disorders too. According to statistics from the National Eating Disorders Association, Black teenagers are 50 percent more likely than white teenagers to exhibit bulimic behavior, such as binging and purging. However, people of color with self-acknowledged eating and weight concerns were significantly less likely than white participants to have been asked by a doctor about eating disorder symptoms, despite similar rates of eating disorder symptoms across ethnic groups.

Additionally, when presented with identical case studies demonstrating disordered eating symptoms in white, Hispanic, and Black women, clinicians were asked to identify if the woman's eating behavior was problematic. Forty-four percent identified the white woman's behavior as problematic, 41 percent identified the Hispanic woman's behavior as problematic, and only 17 percent identified the Black woman's behavior as problematic. The clinicians were also less likely to recommend that the Black woman should receive professional help.

Ultimately, the strength I found in the gym empowered me to join the wellness profession, then use my voice to create change within the industry—to change the landscape of the wellness industry today. And while I may be the one giving talks about these issues and posting about them on social media, I don't believe that my experience is all that unique or different. In fact, I believe that a majority of people, women in particular, struggle with body image issues—which is probably why you're reading this book. We find ourselves trapped and bound by ideas of how we think our bodies are supposed to look and be and unintentionally find ourselves pouring countless amounts of energy into trying to "fix" ourselves.

According to a recent study from Common Sense Media, 80 percent of ten-year-old girls have been on a diet. Furthermore, this "horrifying new research" found that more than half of girls and one-third of boys ages six to eight want thinner bodies. Indeed, these statistics are truly horrifying, but they are far from new. In 1970, the average age a girl began dieting was fourteen, according to the Eating Disorder Foundation. By 1990, that age had dropped to eight. Twenty-five years later, the numbers haven't significantly changed. Each new study on children, dieting, and body image reveals only more appalling details.

This is even more nuanced for those living in Black bodies. In a 2015 study published in the *Journal of Black Psychology*, the authors note that

> *in the past and still today, Black women's bodies and beauty have largely been devalued and rejected by mainstream culture, which overvalues the European aesthetic and undervalues the [aesthetic] of other racial/ethnic [groups] with [the] exception of exoticizing them. The United States puts a premium on "fair" white skin, blue eyes, and long, straight blond hair and considers these features the epitome of beauty. Features more akin to the African [aesthetic] are deemed ugly, undesirable, and less feminine. The notion that Black women are less attractive is a message that is transmitted daily and from multiple external forces and social institutions (e.g., church, government, business industries, media,*

and family and peer groups). Body image and beauty among African American women can be truly under-stood only within a framework of interlocking systems of "isms" (e.g., racism, sexism, classism, heterosexism).

While it's challenging for everyone, it's even more com-plicated for those living in marginalized bodies, as the paper proves. But as my own experience and research have shown, there's something we can do about it. There is a solution. And as you're about to read, *the solution isn't body acceptance or even body positivity.* Those may be an im-portant part of the journey, but the answer . . . is, instead, body liberation, with the recognition that none of us are free unless *all of us are free.*

In the words of Audre Lorde, "I am not free while any woman is unfree, even when her shackles are very differ-ent from my own. And I am not free as long as one person of Color remains chained. Nor is any one of you."

And while Audre Lorde can do absolutely no wrong in my eyes, I like to replace the word "woman" with "person" and the word "her" with "their" because liberation is not bound by gender. It's for everyone.

Our liberation is bound in one another,
and the same is true for our bodies.

The feelings most of us struggle with regarding our bodies often start in our adolescence, and if we never take the time to heal, they can remain with us throughout the duration of our lives. The more energy we spend focusing on shrinking ourselves and conforming to arbitrarily created standards of beauty, the less energy we have to focus on doing our life's work. To being our most true, authentic selves and leaving our mark on the world. We can spend the entirety of our human existence attempting to manufacture ourselves into a "better" version, or we can free ourselves. We can seek liberation.

The reality is that our bodies are constantly changing, and they will never remain exactly the same. If we base our self-worth on something as ever-changing as our bodies, we will forever be on the emotional roller coaster of body obsession and body shame. We are inherently worthy because we exist, not because of what we look like. Developing the ability to radically accept our bodies and recognize their value regardless of how they look is paramount if we ever want to feel at home and at peace with ourselves.

This book is about just that. It's about finding actual freedom in our bodies. It's about understanding that the goal is not to look at our bodies and love everything that we see. It's to understand that at our essence we are so much more than our physical bodies. And it's also about recognizing the harsh realities that prohibit some people from being able to do that as easily.

In 2020, with the murders of George Floyd, Breonna Taylor, and Ahmaud Arbery, we saw social media and the wellness industry spring into action, finally and suddenly waking up to the realities of racism in this country. Black squares of solidarity popped up on social media, and suddenly everyone was interested in diversity and inclusion. While the intention may have been good, in many ways it was self-serving and performative in nature. Performative allyship is harmful to body liberation and collective liberation because it doesn't actually do the work of dismantling. It's simply done to increase a person's or an organization's social capital. It allows you to look good and also feel good without actual devotion to the cause. But left in the aftermath of that is everyone still being harmed by systems of oppression.

While diversity and inclusion are important,
it's often the Band-Aid to actual body liberation.

The reality is that liberation takes real work, a commitment to change, and the willingness to cede power. Ceding power often feels like oppression to individuals who are accustomed to privilege and power. The talk of diversity and inclusion is the easy part. The work required is much harder. Often this is the part people never get to.

In reality, diversity and inclusion are often roadblocks to actual liberation—especially body liberation—because this is the place where the conversation stops. People take the courses and webinars and read the books and believe they have "done the work." But reading is not the work of anti-racism. The work of anti-racism is an ongoing action in our daily lives. Understanding and doing the work of anti-racism is absolutely necessary to body liberation, particularly when the goal is *collective liberation*. So many of our ideals about our bodies are rooted in white supremacy. As we do the work of anti-racism in our lives, we also decolonize our ideas about our bodies.

It took me a long time to unpack the realities of racism and white supremacy and their impact on my ability to love myself wholly and unapologetically. It's nuanced, and I'm still unpeeling layers of the onion. There's no quick five-step process to loving your body. It's not as simple as looking in the mirror and saying positive affirmations to yourself, as body positivity would sometimes lead you to believe. We can't possibly unlearn the narratives we have learned about our bodies without delving into white supremacy.

It's through my experiences of being deep in the throes of body dissatisfaction and diet culture, becoming a trainer and coach, breaking up with diet culture, and finally finding body liberation that I hope to lead you on your own journey to find it for yourself. None of this is easy. None of this is comfortable. In fact, it will likely challenge you in ways that feel wildly disconcerting, regardless of your identity. During my own journey, sharing much of this has also felt uncomfortable for me. Speaking truth to power never happens without pushback. However, I'm again empowered by the words of Audre Lorde:

I write for those women who do not speak, for those who do not have a voice because they were so terrified, because we are taught to respect fear more than our-selves. We've been taught that silence would save us, but it won't.

Silence won't save you. Remaining complicit won't save us. The only way for collective liberation is through dismantling the current systems. And so, this is my contribution toward doing just that. Until we collectively work to dismantle white supremacy and systems of oppression, we are always going to be using Band-Aid approaches to healing our relationships with our bodies. That's not to say we shouldn't use Band-Aids to stop the bleeding. We should, and I do. But we have to go beyond that.

The goal is that once we move toward *personal liberation*, we take that energy and work toward *collective liberation*. We work to change the narrative so those coming after us don't have to fight against the same harmful effects. So our sons and daughters might be born into a kinder, more gentle society—one that nourishes liberation for all.

Have you ever found yourself wondering any of the following?

How do I learn to love and accept my body in a society that tells me everything about my body is wrong?

How is self-love even possible if my body doesn't meet the right "standards"?

Why do I look like this? Why am I not thinner? Prettier? More disciplined?

How can someone in a body like mine feel worthy?

Have you ever had any of the following thoughts?

My life would be so much better if I just lost _____ pounds.

I'll be happy when I can fit comfortably into my old clothes.

I wish I saw myself more represented in fitness and wellness spaces.

I'm tired of seeing the body positivity space co-opted by thin, non-disabled white women.

I'm frustrated that the wellness industry doesn't address racism and white supremacy.

Then you are in the right place. This book is written to set us all free. For us to find freedom in our bodies and seek collective liberation for all.

It's to understand that, at our essence, we are so much more than our bodies.

It's for those of us who have found ourselves on the margins.

It's for anyone seeking liberation.

My desire is that you finish this book feeling emboldened to embrace the body you have now—emboldened to embrace it without condition and to embrace it in all its iterations. I want you to walk away with liberation on your mind—for yourself and for all of us. In the words of my friend Joel Leon, "If it's not about our collective liberation—meaning freedom for ALL of us—I don't want it."

I hope that you don't just read this book and forget about its contents. I sincerely hope that you embody the concepts in this book. To aid you in that, each chapter ends with a section entitled "From Principle to Practice," which serves as guided journal questions, specifically designed to help you internalize the material. To get the most out of this book, I encourage you to take your time going through these questions and journal prompts with thoughtfulness and intention.

From Principle to Practice

———

1. What is your current relationship to your body/ body image?

2. When was the first time you were made to believe something was wrong with your body?

3. What is your earliest memory of believing that being thinner was better?

4. Are you still carrying those stories and beliefs with you? If so, how can you begin to release these narratives that no longer serve you?

5. If you're seeking body liberation, what would that actually look and feel like to you?

CHAPTER 1

Understanding the Basic Concepts:
Body Positivity vs. Body Neutrality vs. Body Liberation

I HAVE TO BE HONEST WITH YOU. TALKING ABOUT DIET CULTURE and the intersection of white supremacy—it's really not a simple topic to address. I want to lead with this statement because, to put it mildly, sometimes people get upset when I voice my views. We are going to talk about a lot of things in this book—privilege, white fragility, and racism, among other things—while we talk about body liberation. In my opinion, we can't talk about liberation without discussing those topics. So if you're a member of the dominant group (i.e., if you're white), I want you to buckle up and get comfortable with the feeling of being uncomfortable.

My brilliant friend Shirin Eskandani once said, "Discomfort is where the growth is, it is where the medicine is, it is where the liberation is." And she's right, y'all. Probably a decade ago, maybe a little more, I stepped into a gym for the first time in my adult life with a singular goal, MAKE ME SKINNY, as I've already shared. Literally, that's what I told my first-ever trainer: I need to be skinny. I was going for the whole model look, you know? I envisioned the end product to be something like Naomi Campbell or Tyra Banks perhaps. You get the vibe. But anyway, before I hired my actual trainer, I did a free session with a male trainer. It was a promotional thing offered by the gym to encourage people to sign up with trainers. Because I went on to get certified and become a trainer myself, I can now confidently say that this man was an awful trainer. Not like he suggested bad exercises or didn't know anything about fitness. No, like he tried to kill me in my free session. I'm serious, y'all. Imagine a novice coming into the gym, bright-eyed and bushy-tailed with false hopes of someday looking like Iman. I was clearly delusional. This man took me through the most intense and challenging workout of my entire life—think lots of jumping, lunging, every high-intensity movement you can imagine. It was my first day in the gym—why would he do that to me? In all fairness, the details are hazy. I don't even remember it all because I almost blacked out. Seriously, I'm not kidding or exaggerating. I started shaking intensely and getting extremely dizzy. So much so that they brought me sugar packets to eat immediately. It was horrible, and yet I still signed up for a trainer—not him, but still, I signed up. The pain of that initial workout didn't deter me enough to quit. Apparently, I'm a glutton for punishment. I later went on to fall in love with strength training and powerlifting, so it was all worth it, despite the rocky start.

What I'm saying is that we have all done some hard things before. So like Shirin says, "If you can understand why the discomfort of a yoga pose is beneficial to your healing and growth, then you must understand that the discomfort of anti-racism work is one and the same." You can replace yoga with any difficult endeavor that you have done in your life. You dealt with the discomfort because you knew something beautiful was on the other side. The same applies as you read this book. If you find yourself feeling triggered or indignant at something I'm discussing, I'm going to politely request that you not be like Diane. Who is Diane, you ask? Diane is an angry person who sent me an email in response to an article I wrote. I really want to share the email with you verbatim because it's truly ludicrous, but apparently there are rules about these things and I guess I would need Diane's permission to share it. I feel very strongly that she would not in fact grant me permission, so I'll paraphrase it for you. It's truly a shame though, because the original email in its entirety is quite a gem.

Dear Miss King,

I have no choice but to email you about your hatred toward white women after receiving a text message about you. I'm going to be honest with you and your entire race, although I know you aren't ready for the truth. Your article is stupid and it's clear that you both hate white women and are jealous of them at the same time. You don't know anything about politics and no one cares what Black people think. Please get over your Black people victim sob story. Everyone is fed up with it, including the Blacks I know. It's clear you are jealous of white women and our beautiful glowing skin that you will never get to have. But you'll likely say I'm racist—LOLOLOLOL. In the future, you are going to be embarrassed of your conduct. Stop being stupid and find something of substance to write about.

Ciao, Diane

This is the watered-down version of the email, but alas, you get the gist of it. Ahh, Diane. Besides the fact that this email doesn't make sense in a lot of ways, it was also a complete waste of time. I don't reply to emails like this, y'all. So if you find yourself about to pull a Diane, dig out your journal and go "Dear Diary" style instead. Perhaps write out your feelings, and curiously and compassionately consider why you're feeling so triggered. But for the love of God, do not email me.

In the words of Layla Saad, "You cannot dismantle what you cannot see. You cannot challenge what you do not understand." As we work to dismantle diet culture and white supremacy in our lives, it can be an uncomfortable process. It's not warm and fuzzy work, and sometimes it has the potential to feel painful, disconcerting, and triggering. But we gotta face the facts, even when they're not pretty. It's all part of the process. When I first started powerlifting seriously, I developed a power phrase that I would repeat to myself before every heavy lift. "I can do hard things." That phrase served me in the gym and has since become a part of my practice anytime I'm doing something hard, in or out of the gym. I invite you to try it for yourself anytime you feel things getting hard. "I can do hard things." But honestly, if this book found its way to you, I trust that you're reading it because you are ready to embrace the body you have right now, and because you want liberation for yourself, and for all of us. Okay, so now that we got that out of the way, let's dive in.

While the words "body positivity," "body neutrality," and "body liberation" are often used interchangeably, in my opinion, they are quite different. It's wholly necessary that we understand the difference between these terms and truthfully interrogate the problems with some of these spaces.

If you do a simple Google search asking the question "What is body positivity?" you will get an array of answers, but most of them describe body positivity as a movement focused on empowering individuals to love and appreciate their bodies regardless of their size, shape, or weight. It preaches that all bodies are worthy of respect and love. If you look at the hashtag #BodyPositivity on Instagram, you will likely see a lot of women wearing swimsuits and discussing how much they love their bodies despite the fact that society has tried to tell them something was wrong with their bodies. You will probably also see a lot of messages about self-love mixed into the discussion.

While I think body positivity can be a good introduction to the concept of thinking about our bodies differently, I also believe that mainstream body positivity, now popular and trendy on social media outlets such as Instagram, can often prove to be a double-edged sword. Yes, in a lot of ways it can be helpful and has absolutely encouraged millions of people to feel better about their relationships with their bodies, but it's also been unintentionally harmful as well.

A lot of the messaging in the body positivity space encourages us to just love our bodies. If you have ever been on the receiving end of these messages, perhaps you found them frustrating. I know I did at times. If everyone else was capable of just donning a swimsuit and falling in love with their bodies, why wasn't I? The affirmations and mantras you were supposed to repeat to yourself didn't seem to be so effective when I tried them. I can't even tell you the amount of times I looked in the mirror repeating affirmations to myself only to walk away discouraged and frustrated with the image I saw reflected back.

If you're deep in the trenches grappling with body

image issues, and you're being inundated with body positive influencers preaching self-love, all now appearing to effortlessly love their bodies, it can feel extremely frustrating. To be honest, telling people to just "love their bodies" isn't that helpful. If it were that easy, wouldn't we all already be doing that? And if you are already struggling with body image, watching other people pop the words "body positivity" on captions, encouraging you to just embrace yourself when that feels like the furthest thing from possible, often leaves you swimming in more guilt and shame. Here is another thing you have failed at. Everyone has found a way to accept their bodies, but you can't even do that.

While the movement largely focuses on self-love, it largely fails to acknowledge that it's much easier for some individuals to love themselves than for others. In a society in which certain bodies are deemed more beautiful, more worthy of dignity and respect, and, honestly, more valuable, I would argue that body positivity shouldn't just be about loving your body. It should be demanding justice for all bodies, especially the most marginalized. The intersection of race, gender, body politics, age, sexual orientation, and ability status are often left out of the conversation about body positivity. If social justice isn't at the core of the movement, there's nothing really radical about it, and it definitely isn't helping people find liberation.

While self-love and empowering individuals to appreciate their bodies are certainly part of it, the reality is that the body positivity movement has its roots in the fat acceptance movement of the 1960s, and it was created as a safe space for fat women and Black women to celebrate themselves and accept their bodies as beautiful in a world where they didn't see that reflected. It was really created for those on the margins of mainstream ideals of beauty—think Black and brown bodies, fat bodies, disabled bodies, trans bodies, etc. It was also rooted in social justice. However, mainstream body positivity has lost its focus in a lot of ways and has been co-opted and whitewashed, including even the history of the movement, with many individuals crediting plus-size model Tess Holliday, who is white, as the movement's creator because of a popular #EffYour BeautyStandards hashtag she started in 2013.

As Stephanie Yeboah, freelance writer and author of *Fattily Ever After: A Black Fat Girl's Guide to Living Life Unapologetically*, says, "[Body positivity] stems from the fat acceptance movement, which is more political than anything, [and] was created as a safe space for fat women to celebrate themselves as no one was celebrating us or seeing us—and all our interior amazingness—for what we were. Now it's used as a marketing term and has forgotten about the very bodies that created it."

The faces of body positivity have largely become thinner, straight-sized (a term used to describe the clothing sizes used by most designers, typically below a size 10), cisgender, non-disabled white women discussing embracing their rolls and cellulite. The issue is more than just the fact that they fail to acknowledge the origin of the movement—they also fail to realize how they take up too much space, pushing out the very individuals who created the movement. Now that body positivity has become commercialized and profitable, these individuals are also able to profit financially off the labor of Black, brown, and fat people. Think Instagram ads, campaigns, and modeling jobs for companies that want to be body positive, and the majority of the individuals getting these opportunities are white women, not fat Black and brown women.

In a 2017 article for *Elle*, Yeboah states, "Arguably, much like the feminist movement, body positivity has become non-intersectional and prioritises/celebrates the thoughts, feelings, opinions and achievements of white women, with a small number of 'token' people of colour to help fill up the 'look at us being diverse!' quota."

Lizzo, who has had her fair share of body critique over the years, took to social media to voice her critique of the body positive movement. "Because now that body positivity has been co-opted by all bodies and people are finally celebrating medium and small girls and people who occasionally get rolls, fat people are still getting the short end of this movement. . . . It's like, 'Body positivity is for everybody.' Yes, please be positive about your body. Please use our movement to empower yourself. That's the point! But the people who created this movement—big women, big brown and Black women, queer women—are not benefiting from the mainstream success of it."

Social media has always been a place where I share snippets of my work and thoughts that I have. I talked about this topic on Instagram in a post stating,

Mainstream body positivity misses the mark. A movement created by Black women has unfortunately been co-opted by thinner, white women taking pictures of themselves in the mirror showing a few stretch marks, a tad of cellulite, or arched over to display a bit of tummy fat. These individuals, often attractive by Eurocentric standards of beauty, perhaps well-intentioned, are often misguided and disregard the history of the movement, failing to recognize the privilege they have from residing in a body that is already very close to idealized standards. Even more, they fail to recognize that their ability to be the poster children of the self-love/body positive movement is still rooted in white supremacy. The current state of body positivity focuses on self-love often without acknowledging that it's much easier for some individuals than others, disregarding the intersection of race, gender, body politics, sexual orientation, and ability status. I argue that body positivity isn't about just loving your body. It should be about demanding justice for all bodies, especially the most marginalized.

I went on to say that I encourage us all (myself included) to think critically about the ways in which we may be participating in systems of oppression and being complicit within them. While I'm beginning to see more people acknowledging the problems, what 1 don't see as often is changed behavior. Choosing to engage in something that you acknowledge is problematic because it benefits you is still continued participation in white supremacy.

The comments section (and the post) went wild. Here are a few of my favorite comments:

Omg how self involved can you be. Body positivity is about loving your body whether or not it is fat OR skinny, brown OR not totally brown, or whatever YOU see in the mirror that bothers you that you feel you should accept. Rooted in white supremacy? Girl that's a stretch and a half. Putting down white girls just tryna accept themselves too to make you feel better is all you've said here. And it's really ridiculous.

So thin white women are not welcome in the movement and can't feel bad about their bodies and if they do it's rooted in white supremacy?? If this is the case when creating a movement a clear mission and [who] is and isn't allowed to participate should be made known. But I do wonder if a movement was made by a thinner white woman and said sorry this doesn't apply to large black women—they would be shunned and called racist? Division is created and anytime division is created more issues and hate arises and that's not what we need right now.

I'm sorry, what was the point of this? White, asian, indeed any non-black person with image issues and body acceptance issues is now being told to what, continue the shame cycle they put upon themselves in order to only let one kind of person own the monopoly over a movement which was intended to elevate and bring joy to millions of suffering individuals? I mean this in the best way, but self image is rooted in more than just "Eurocentric" beauty standards. There are more races than just black and white. Please tell any of the painfully anorexic Asian women who starve their already frail bodies into submission to look more like celebrities in their countries, or Jewish girls who feel the need to get nose surgeries and painful laser surgeries to rid themselves of physical attributes which far outstrip their whiteness when it comes to self confidence. It is very upsetting that you feel only fat black women should be visible members of a self-love movement.

Y'all, did this last individual actually say "tell any of the painfully anorexic Asian women who starve their already frail bodies into submission"?! Yes. Yes, indeed, that was said. I won't say the race or ethnicity of this person, but I will say that they were not Asian.

Sometimes I get frustrated with social media because, alas, it appears people don't read. Please go back to my original statement. Which part of my post said that white women can't suffer from body image issues? Which part of my post said that white women couldn't be involved in the body positivity space? Which part of my post said that only fat Black women should be visible members of the movement?

The responses highlighted above are peak white fragility mixed with a healthy dose of white feminism. "White fragility," a term coined by Robin DiAngelo in her book *White Fragility*, is defined as a state in which "the smallest amount of racial stress is intolerable—the mere suggestion that being white has meaning often triggers a range of defensive responses." "Feminism," according to *Merriam-Webster*, is defined as "a range of socio-political movements and ideologies that aim to define and establish the political, economic, personal, and social equality of the sexes," or as "the advocacy of women's rights on the basis of gender equality." "White feminism," broadly defined by Wikipedia, is "a term used to describe expressions of feminism which are perceived as focusing on the struggles of white women while failing to address distinct forms of oppression faced by ethnic minority women and women lacking other privileges."

Whenever I hear a white woman use the word "divisive" when race is being discussed, I already know their white fragility is showing. It shows up as defensiveness, tone policing, accusing people of sowing division, victim blaming, or taking on the role of the victim when someone is pointing out problematic or racist behavior, even if it's not about them directly. Instead of being able to listen to a critique and consider the validity, white folks make it about themselves and their feelings. And for a lot of white folks, being called racist, or the insinuation that their behavior is racist or rooted in white supremacy, is the worst insult you could possibly bestow upon them. Austin Channing Brown, author of *I'm Still Here: Black Dignity in a World Made for Whiteness*, discusses this phenomenon in her book, stating, "White people desperately want to believe that only the lonely, isolated 'whites only' club members are racist. This is why the word *racist* offends 'nice white people' so deeply. It challenges their self-identification as good people. Sadly, most white people are more worried about being called racist than about whether or not their actions are in fact racist or harmful."

The thing that is so jarring about white feminism is that feminism is about the equality of the sexes. So in that sense, it's easy for white women to recognize when there are inequalities present that are based on gender and that personally affect them. But on the flip side, they have a difficult time seeing the implications of race and racism as it pertains to Black and brown women. It's easy to say that the patriarchy is responsible for our body image issues, because that puts much of the blame on men, but it's often far more difficult to point to white supremacy as the culprit, because that doesn't absolve white women of their participation in the system.

When I call out the problems with the mainstream body positivity space and the ways in which some white women within the space are complicit with the system of white supremacy, outrage often ensues. Instead of thinking critically about how members of the dominant group are taking up too much space, colonizing, taking over—or whatever you want to call it—a space that was created by others to center the experiences of those in historically underrepresented and oppressed bodies, white feminism wants to continue centering their own experiences and pain. White supremacy and white feminism are barriers to collective body liberation. White feminism willfully ignores the experiences of Black women and women of color, particularly when it challenges or requires changed behavior from white women.

I realize that it's pretty popular to display your body—imperfections and all—in pictures for social media and talk about body positivity. And to be fair, I think it's helpful for all humanity to see all different types of bodies represented on mainstream platforms. But we cannot pretend that the repercussions of having a tiny bit of cellulite are the same as experiencing serious weight stigma for living in a fat body. In addition, the things we often characterize as flaws—cellulite, body hair, hip dips, belly rolls, stretch marks—aren't imperfections or flaws at all. They are simple natural occurrences for any of us having this human experience. It's just a body being a body.

Jessie Mundell, an online exercise coach for pregnancy, postpartum, and parents, speaks of her role as a white coach in the online space: "Showing an image of grabbing a handful of belly fat on your white body isn't radical." Jessie goes on to say that she is not a body positive fitness trainer, specifically because the work of body positivity was born from Black women and femmes: "My role within this is to amplify and centre the voices of those people."

I have to agree with Jessie. It's simply not radical. There's nothing brave about posting a picture of yourself as a thin to medium-sized, white, cisgender, non-disabled person on the internet, even if there is a bit of cellulite, acne, or body fat. I don't know how else to say this, but that's about as normal as a body can get. I'm not saying these folks shouldn't post their pictures, but I am suggesting that perhaps it should not be done under the guise of body positivity.

There have been a myriad of discussions about this matter in the online body positivity space as individuals attempt to be more "woke" and supposedly disavow white supremacy, especially after summer 2020, when white folks suddenly awoke to the realities of racism. Many white influencers who have been called out for co-opting the body positivity space are now attempting to shy away from use of the term or to explain their privilege as a footnote to the work they are putting out.

What I see occurring is that individuals who have built a platform (and sometimes, even an entire career) off co-opting the body positivity space are now, after being called out or perhaps becoming educated about the roots of the body positivity space, attempting to rectify their mistakes without actually doing what that requires—thus not actually rectifying anything at all. The reality is that once you understand the problematic nature of profiting from a space that was never created for you, the only way to actually rectify it is to remove yourself from the space—to actively take up less space. However, that would also require that you give up certain opportunities and, ultimately, probably money as well.

And here's where the rubber meets the road. Most people are willing to disavow white supremacy in words and deeds but not necessarily in action. It's easy to say that something is bad, but it's much harder to part ways when you feel like it will cost you something. The reality is individuals like the privileges that white supremacy affords them. Within the realm of the body positivity space that means the ability to land campaigns, speaking opportunities, and make money. You simply can't do both. You can't acknowledge the issues and at the same time continue to participate because it benefits you. Because it affords you a lifestyle that you enjoy. When you willingly participate even though you know the problems, you are complicit, and white supremacy thrives off the complicit individual. All this means is that people love their comfort and personal liberation more than the collective.

Unfortunately, when it comes to dismantling white supremacy, a lot of folks do choose themselves (and their privilege) over the collective. Likewise, a lot of folks aren't really interested in justice and equity for all bodies. A lot of folks are interested in their individual ability to succeed as a primary focus, and are only interested in dismantling systems if it doesn't affect them personally, especially as it pertains to capitalism. Dismantling comes at a price. It will also cost something, and it always requires sacrifice.

If you fail to acknowledge the ways in which the body positivity movement continues to center white women and allows them opportunities that members of historically excluded communities—think BIPOC (Black, Indigenous, people of color), 2SLGBTQIA+ folks, and disabled folks— don't have access to, it's shallow and shortsighted. There is no dismantling or liberation without sacrifice. If you can name the issues with the space but are unwilling to pass up opportunities, money, and relationships to demand justice and equity (including financial equity) for all bodies, then you aren't doing the work of body positivity and definitely not of liberation. The anti-diet movement must be firmly rooted in social justice and dismantling systems of oppression in order to work toward collective liberation.

I want to be really clear about something. Everyone, regardless of size, shape, ethnicity, or identity, can have a hard time loving their body, and to be fair, a lot of us struggle with embracing and accepting ourselves. It's not just Black women or folks in larger bodies. Because we have all been indoctrinated in a patriarchal society hyperfocused on western standards of beauty, we are all, women in particular, at greater risk for body image issues. However, the terms "body positivity" and "body image" are often conflated. It's important that we have a clear understanding of how these things differ as we seek to fully understand body positivity. "Body image," as defined by the National Eating Disorders Association, "is how you see yourself when you look in the mirror or when you picture yourself in your mind."

It encompasses:
- *What you believe about your own appearance (including your memories, assumptions, and generalizations).*
- *How you feel about your body, including your height, shape, and weight.*
- *How you sense and control your body as you move. How you physically experience or feel in your body.*

When we think about body image, it's really about how we think about ourselves. Our relationship with our body image has absolutely been influenced by life experiences, most likely starting from early childhood. Our relationship to our body image has been impacted by the way our parents and familial units spoke about their bodies, the way our peers speak about their bodies, the media we consume, and a variety of other messages we receive about what the "ideal" or desirable body is.

When I say that the body positivity space is being

co-opted, it doesn't mean that white women can't have body image issues or discuss their struggles with body image. Of course they can. However, it's important that we distinguish between having a personal struggle with body image and facing systemic oppression or discrimination *because* of your body. Those are two wildly different experiences, and it's important to acknowledge and understand the difference between these two scenarios.

Looking in the mirror and being at war with the reflection, whether it be because of cellulite, stretch marks, belly rolls, or any of the other completely normal body attributes that we have been made to believe are "flaws," is hard as hell. Obsessing about your body will literally drain you mentally and physically. It divests us of our personal power because every part of our life is overshadowed by being uncomfortable in our skin. None of us are immune from this experience.

However, overt discrimination and weight stigma are completely different beasts. Not being able to fit into an airplane seat or into a booth at a restaurant because the world caters to thinness as a norm is not only a weight stigma but is also actual oppression. The experience of living in a Black body or a fat body or a trans body is not the same as being dissatisfied with what you see in the mirror. And this is the crucial difference that everyone frustrated by my post doesn't tend to understand. The body positivity space was created by fat Black women as a space to celebrate themselves because the world didn't. Now it centers white women, and therein lies the problem. It's not a problem for white women to find the body positivity movement helpful for their journey with body acceptance. It's a problem when the movement caters to and centers them.

I deeply empathize with every single person who has ever felt (or still feels) utterly miserable because of the body they reside in. It's important to me that you understand how sincerely I mean that. I hold so much compassion for all of us because body shit is hard. Really hard. We likely can all recall instances that have made us feel insecure about our bodies or our looks. In her book *The Body Is Not an Apology: The Power of Radical Self-Love*, Sonya Renee Taylor speaks of the concept of body shame origin stories—describing the first memory we have of body shame. The moment when someone led us to believe there was something wrong with us or made us feel insecure about ourselves. We all have these memories.

I have so many it's hard to choose, but I'll share one about something that is deeply personal to many Black women—our hair.

The year is 1996. I'm nine years old. I'm attending a small Christian school, Calvary Baptist, in the suburbs in Wisconsin. There are only a handful of students of color, probably eight at most (two of those being my brother and sister), and no other Black kids. To add even more context to this story, this is my first time attending school with other kids, because I was homeschooled until the third grade. My mom educated my siblings and me at home before shipping us off to a private school, where I was required to attend chapel each week and wear skirts that covered my knees. Did my parents want to torture me? I wonder about that myself sometimes, but ultimately, I think they believed they were giving us the best opportunities they could provide and hopefully setting us up for success.

I made friends easily. My class had only twenty kids in it, so it really wasn't that difficult. But being the only Black girl made the experience interesting, especially considering none of my classmates had previously had any Black friends. This was the kind of school where the girls in the class all invited each other to sleep over at their homes. Sleepovers were still somewhat new to me. My mom was strict, and it's just not something we did, because she was not having it. My parents kept us at home, where they could keep their eyes on us. But somehow, once we started attending this school, they began loosening up and allowing us to stay over at friends' houses. I had a lot of sleepovers during this time—most of them I have no recollection of. But there are two sleepovers in particular that are etched into my brain. I'm going to tell you about one of them now. You know how Black women have entire songs dedicated to people not touching our hair? Cue Solange's "Don't Touch My Hair." Well, there's a valid reason for this. I was at one of my first sleepovers at a classmate's house, and someone asked to play in my hair. Now, the grown-ass Chrissy of today will literally swat away the hand of anyone who dares to come near my mane (and I have had to do this too many times to count in my adult life), but nine-year-old Chrissy replied, "Sure." The next thing I know, my friend has unbraided one of my pigtails and is caressing my hair, followed quickly by shrieking, "Eww gross. Why does it feel greasy? When was the last time you washed your hair? And why does it feel so hard?"

As you can imagine, I was embarrassed and ashamed. And to make matters worse, then everyone else wanted to feel it, only to come to the same conclusion. I literally wanted to disappear. I had already felt different prior to this moment. I was tall and Black in a world filled with average-height girls with blond and brunette hair. And thus began my complicated relationship with my hair, which would last through my twenties.

So you know what I did to compensate? For starters, I insisted that I get a perm. For Black people, a perm is a process that chemically straightens your hair. I wanted long, flowing, silky locs like my peers, not the kinky and coily hair that naturally grew from my scalp. Next, I stopped putting moisture in my hair. For the Black women reading this book, do you remember Ultra Sheen hair grease? It's the super-thick blue hair grease that our moms used to religiously grease our scalps with. Well, I forsook Ultra Sheen because I really just didn't want to be different. Obviously, Black hair needs moisture, probably not Ultra Sheen—but listen, our moms were doing their best. As a result, my hair got so dry that one day I was brushing my bangs and kept noticing flakes flying. At first, I thought it was dandruff flakes, but to my horror, I realized that it was actually my hair breaking off in tiny pieces because it was so dry and brittle. That was a wake-up call. I could try as hard as I wanted to be like the little white girls in my class; my hair didn't give one fuck about that. Needless to say, I added some moisture back to my hair-care routine after that.

That's one of my body shame stories. If you're not Black, you may not quite understand what my hair has to do with my body. For many Black women, myself included, hair is deeply tied to our identities. It's tradition. It's a form of self-expression. It's culture. On many levels, it's just as much who we are as our bodies. When your hair has been constantly questioned, demonized, and touched by non-melanated strangers on the streets, trust me, it's part of your story.

Beyond that, many of us with kinky, coily, and curly hair have had to face actual repercussions for our tresses—from simply being told our hair looks "unkempt" to job discrimination. For those who are unfamiliar, hair discrimination is a very real thing, with only fourteen states across the United States having put laws into place to ban Black hair discrimination. Yes, there are still thirty-six states in the US of A that don't protect Black folks from facing discrimination for how they choose to wear their hair. Anti-discrimination laws to protect Black folks and our hair are necessary because in 2018, eleven-year-old Faith Fennidy was sent home from school in tears for having braids, as the school had implemented a policy that "only the students' natural hair is permitted," and also in 2018, Andrew Johnson, a Black wrestler, was forced to cut his dreadlocks in order to compete in his match.

Our body shame stories play a key role in the development of our body image. It sets the foundation as we reach adolescence, and many of us are still carrying these painful stories and memories with us in adulthood. What about you? What's your body shame story? What is the memory, or memories, that stands out in your mind that shaped your body image?

I firmly believe that every single person reading this has a story, and your story is real and valid. Your experiences are real and valid. If you have suffered from body dysmorphia or eating disorders or just spent the majority of your life uncomfortable in your skin, I am not in any way minimizing that experience. I'm simply asking you to consider that sometimes members of the dominant group actually need to take up less space in certain circumstances, especially within spaces that weren't created with them in mind, like the body positivity space.

MOVING BEYOND BODY POSITIVITY, WE HAVE "BODY NEUTRALITY," a term coined and popularized in 2015, which seeks to help us come to a place where we can be neutral with ourselves. It's essentially about coming to a place of acceptance with the current state of our bodies. We don't necessarily love our bodies, but we choose not to speak about our bodies with disdain and hate. We choose not to put ourselves down, even when we don't feel good about our bodies. We can begin to show our bodies respect and appreciation for all they allow us to do, even if we don't necessarily like everything about them. It can also mean choosing not to even think much about our bodies, one way or the other. We just exist and allow our bodies to be and respect them, without giving them too much thought.

As you noticed, the title of this book is *The Body Liberation Project*, so it's clear that I want all of us to experience liberation. However, going from body shame to liberation is a canyon far too wide for most of us to leap over. The body positivity space often offers the advice to state positive affirmations such as "I love my body" and "My body is perfect just as it is." While I believe affirmations can be a powerful tool for changing our mindset, often there is also an element of false positivity. I've said this earlier in the chapter, but I think it's worth repeating: If you are experiencing an extremely negative body image, telling yourself that you love your body probably isn't the thing that's actually going to help move the needle. Instead of being inauthentic about how we feel about our bodies, neutrality offers the opportunity to meet ourselves with acceptance. Body neutrality is more attainable as a first step toward liberation, while we work toward finding our own personal freedom in our bodies. Instead of looking in the mirror and immediately telling ourselves we look gross, maybe we can look in the mirror and simply acknowledge, "This is how my body looks today," without making any disparaging comments.

Even still, we have to consider the implication of intersecting identities and the impact that has on one's ability to practice body neutrality or even acceptance. When an individual has been faced with the challenges of fatphobia, ableism, and anti-Blackness, among other things, it's easy to see why even being neutral about your body can be a huge feat when you are constantly inundated with messages that tell you otherwise. Additionally, for individuals faced with physical disabilities, it can feel difficult to even be neutral about your body when you feel like it has betrayed you in some way. I myself have been guilty of saying things like "Focus on what your body can do instead of what it looks like," without acknowledging the ableist nature of that statement or even the privilege of existing as a person without disabilities.

But regardless of this, I think we deserve more than to just be neutral or accept our bodies. Not that there's anything wrong with neutrality—I just want us all to unapologetically and unabashedly cherish ourselves. I believe the thing we are seeking is liberation. By definition, "liberation" means the act of setting someone free from imprisonment, slavery, or oppression. Tina Strawn, author of *Are We Free Yet? The Black Queer Guide to Divorcing America*, describes liberation as "a celebration of our deepest humanity, and our fight for it must include a deeper examination of how we relate to oppressive systems while centering our joy, peace, and pleasure." This quote embodies the essence of body liberation. It's about understanding the systems that would have us at war with ourselves, while learning to embrace joy and pleasure in ourselves. Unfortunately, so many of us have become imprisoned to unrealistic ideals about bodies. But we are the ones we have been waiting for. We are setting ourselves free. Because life is too short to spend our entire existence obsessing about our bodies and trying to shrink ourselves, physically and metaphorically.

When we achieve body liberation, we realize that our bodies are the least interesting thing about us. It's about understanding that the goal is not to look at our bodies and love everything that we see. It's to understand that at our essence we are so much more than our bodies. They are simply the vessels that allow us to have this human experience. We can spend the entirety of our human existence attempting to manufacture ourselves into a better version—or we can be free ourselves.

But it is also about recognizing the hard realities that prohibit people from being able to do that. The goal is not just to find your own personal body liberation and move on with your life, happy and free. The end goal is a world where every *body* is free to exist, free from harm, discrimination, and harassment. The goal is freedom for everyone, especially those with multiple intersecting identities. In the words of American civil rights activist Fannie Lou Hamer, "Nobody's free until everybody's free."

Body liberation goes beyond body positivity, body neutrality, body acceptance, self-love, and any of the other phrases we have adapted to talk about fostering a healthy relationship with our bodies. The goal of liberation is that we can reclaim all the time, energy, and emotion we have put into yearning for the "perfect" body and find actual freedom. I don't want us to just accept or be neutral about bodies. Yes, we will likely go through that stage on the way to liberation, but do we really want to tolerate our "imperfections," or can we decolonize our minds so that we realize our "imperfections" aren't flaws at all? They're simply the normal experience of having a body.

So going back to my earlier story and my difficult relationship with my hair. I could have spent the rest of my life wishing my hair were different. That my curls were looser. That my locs were more flowy. But again, what a waste of time it would have been wishing for what I couldn't change. Instead, I finally decided to embrace what was growing naturally out of my scalp. I don't remember what led me to the decision. I don't remember exactly what I was thinking, but one day, it just clicked. This time cue India.Arie's "I Am Not My Hair." I was twenty-one years old, and I decided I wanted to get rid of all my permed hair and start over. I went to the hair salon and got a big chop, which is just a phrase to describe the process of cutting off your chemically straightened hair to let it grow in its natural texture. And I set about the journey of falling in love with my hair all over again. Learning to embrace my hair was a step toward liberation.

As I close out this chapter, I invite you to take some time to think critically about where you are in your own journey toward liberation. Perhaps body positivity introduced you to the realization that you could think differently about your body. I think that's true for a lot of people, and honestly, that's a beautiful thing. While I have expressed my personal opinions about the shortcomings of the body positivity space, I also acknowledge that despite some of the issues, it's invited so many of us to interrogate the messages we've been force-fed about our bodies and perhaps has led us on a journey of self-exploration.

Maybe you're currently in a space of body neutrality, and you're working to meet yourself with compassion and kindness instead of disdain. I remember being in that place myself, and for me, it was an important part of my journey. The reality is that no one jumps from body shame and hate to liberation. And for many of us, liberation is years in the making.

And finally, maybe you're already in a place of liberation. You feel free in your body. You understand that the way you look is the least interesting thing about you, and you feel so good in your skin. You unabashedly and unapologetically love and honor yourself. I'm so happy for you. This is a beautiful place to be in. And yet, it's a journey that never truly ends. We fight for liberation day after day, always reminding ourselves of what we know to be true.

From Principle to Practice

1. Now that you've learned the difference between body positivity, body neutrality, and body liberation, what stage are you currently in?

2. What implications have race, gender, sexuality, or your ability status had on your relationship with your body?

3. Regardless of the fact that you may not like everything about your body, can you show it love and appreciation despite your current feelings about it?

4. What are one to three ways you can work to meet your body with compassion instead of disdain this week?

5. Write a love note to your body every morning this week.

CHAPTER 2

Why Body Liberation Is Needed:

Educating Yourself about the Historical Roots of the Intersection of Diet Culture and White Supremacy

WHEN I WAS SIXTEEN YEARS OLD, I GOT A JOB AS A CASHIER AT Target, and I was so excited about it. I purchased a few pairs of khakis and red shirts as soon as I got the good news. I felt so lucky to be working there. I mean, who wouldn't want to work at Target?! Even back then, I possessed the same enthusiasm for the store that I have now. The fact that I can't leave the store without spending at least $100, even when I only go in for toothpaste, doesn't deter me. Any excuse is a good reason to go to Target. When I first moved to Brooklyn from Milwaukee, I was a tad disappointed because the Targets here aren't as sprawling as I'm used to, due to the general lack of space. They are fine, but imagine the shock when I realized some of them don't have a shoe section. It's not like I buy a lot of shoes at Target, but I like to have the option. On one of my first visits back home after relocating, I went to my favorite Target—the one sixteen-year-old me worked at—and lost my mind. It was like I had been wandering in the desert for years and was now back in a land flowing with milk and honey. I was so happy to be back in the type of Target I'm used to that I spent almost $600. I was buying anything and everything in sight simply because I could; it was all there. I got so much that I had to ship two boxes of stuff back to Brooklyn. It was like I blacked out.

So what I'm saying is that my love for Target runs deep, and it began many years ago. My time as a cashier preceded self-checkout lines and Apple Pay. In fact, I was working there when chip readers were just becoming a thing, and when Target installed them, we were all in awe of how fancy these new payment systems were. One night we left the store and the next day we had been upgraded. It was pretty cool. We got training and then we also had to show customers how to use the new system to make payments because it was new to all of us. So one day, I'm doing my cashier thing, and a white, middle-aged couple comes to my line. I scanned all their items and told them the total, and when the man proceeded to hand me his credit card for payment, I explained that he could insert it himself now. That man looked me dead in the eye and said, "Wow. They had to make it easier for you people, but I guess you can teach monkeys anything." His wife elbowed him, and he had the audacity to say, "What? I'm just telling the truth." I remained silent, but on the inside, I was angry and frustrated. I finished the transaction and handed the man his receipt, and he said one last thing to me: "You're pretty cute for a Black girl. That's a good thing, especially if your career aspirations are being a cashier. I didn't mean anything racist by the monkey joke. I just mean that people have no skills these days."

I thought about that interaction for many days after that, and I've had many experiences since then that all had the same underlying theme. When I was an undergraduate student at a PWI (predominantly white institution), I had a professor who told me he wasn't going to give me a good grade just because of affirmative action. This was before he even knew anything about me. Later, he gave me an A in that course and told me that I had "surprised him." For the entirety of my life, I've had people make assumptions and judgments about me simply because I reside in a Black body.

"You are more than your body." I've heard this a thousand times, and I say it frequently myself. It's such a nuanced statement. On the one hand, it's absolutely true. We *are* so much more than our bodies. On the other hand, regardless of that, existing in our respective bodies has implications, and the implications are different depending on the body in question. I would bet money that my former professor didn't tell any of his white students he was surprised they had earned As, and I'm also pretty positive he never addressed affirmative action with them.

When we throw around the phrase "more than your body" without acknowledging the social and political implications of our bodies—what living in certain bodies actually means for people's ability to feel safe and secure in their skin—we disregard the way people experience the world. Most simply put, we are all living in a body, but we are all having vastly different experiences. So while it's true that we are all more than our bodies, that doesn't negate the fact that our bodies play a significant role in our lives.

So many of the conversations about bodies focus on self-love as the anecdote to body shame. While I agree that self-love is a worthwhile and necessary endeavor, it doesn't address the realities of living in a white supremacist society that is inherently fatphobic, homophobic, and transphobic, nor does it address the realities of diet culture. The simplest definition of this term is that "diet culture" is a system of beliefs that worships thinness and equates it to health and moral virtue. It convinces us that weight loss and the attainment of a smaller body will make our lives better and "healthier," even though it forces many of us into yo-yo dieting, which has been shown to have a detrimental impact on our health, such as an increased risk of developing heart disease and a greater potential to develop issues with binge eating.

Aside from that, it also oppresses individuals who don't

match up to the arbitrary picture of health, having an even more detrimental impact on women, BIPOC, trans folks, people with disabilities, and folks in larger bodies. Diet culture most certainly wreaks havoc on us all; however, the impact is more severe for some people than others. The hyperfocus on self-love within body positivity fails to address the fact that self-love doesn't change the systemic oppression that one may experience from living in a fat body or a trans body or a Black body. So much of the mainstream body positivity space has now become focused on how we can learn to love our bodies and ourselves in a world that wants us to hate ourselves. While I understand this thought process and the sentiment and wholeheartedly believe that loving ourselves deeply is necessary, I would like to offer to the conversation the reality that all the self-love in the world won't save a person from the western standards of beauty that are rooted in white supremacy and racism. Nor will loving ourselves prevent any of us from experiencing harm in the world or from experiencing systemic discrimination.

Our cultural obsession with thinness, our desire to be thin—no matter the cost—and our incessant desire to pursue that as the status quo stem from the fact that diet culture is heavily rooted in racism and white supremacy. As Sabrina Strings, PhD, discusses in her book, *Fearing the Black Body: The Racial Origins of Fat Phobia*, Black people have historically, and intentionally, been linked with fatness dating as far back as the nineteenth century. "One of the things that the colonists believed was that Black people were inherently more sensuous, people that love sex and they love food, and so the idea was that Black people had more venereal diseases and that Black people were inherently obese because they lack self-control," Strings said in an interview. "And of course, self-control and rationality, after the Enlightenment, were characteristics that were deemed integral to whiteness." Over time, this connection between Black people and gluttony has become internalized and upheld, making diet culture's rejection of larger bodies inherently racist, argues Strings. Connecting fatness to Blackness was a way to not only justify slavery but also deem Black people as inferior to white people. Anti-fat bias and fatphobia are inextricably tied to racism, and even if we don't know or understand the history, our participation in the system is still participation in white supremacy. As Strings said, "We cannot deny the fact that fatphobia is rooted in anti-Blackness. That's simply a historical reality. Today, when people talk about it, they often claim that they don't intend to be anti-Black . . . they don't intend all of these negative associations, and yet they exist already, so whenever people start trafficking in fatphobia, they are inherently picking up on these historical forms of oppression."

Whether we consciously realize it or not, we've all been influenced by diet culture and racism, but the fact that fatphobia has its roots in racism means that the impact of diet culture for those living in Black, larger bodies is even greater. No amount of self-love changes that, and no amount of self-love saves people from the consequences of living in a marginalized body.

My friend Ilya Parker, besides being a brilliant educator, is also the founder of Decolonizing Fitness, a social justice platform that provides affirming fitness services, community education, and apparel in support of body diversity. Being a Black, nonbinary, trans masculine person in a white supremacist society has led them to have a myriad of experiences from which self-love could not save them. As Ilya has told me:

> I can't count how many times I've heard as a trans person: "You just have a body image issue, and if you practice more self-love, you would be okay." Messages like this are often shared by well-meaning people who lack depth around the fact that all bodies are politicized. Meaning, everyone's body is treated a certain way according to their race, gender, size, ability, etc. We are more than just individuals having a lone connection with our bodies. Our bodies are political statements, and depending on which body you are in, it will certainly dictate how society treats you.
>
> Let's unpack "the body is political" a bit by using myself as an example. I identify as and am often read by the world as a Black transgender person who is also fat. Each of those identities is connected to a separately

oppressed population (i.e., Black people, trans people, fat people). These identities of oppression are also intersecting, which often creates exacerbated layers of marginalization for me. Many days I have experienced anti-Black, anti-trans, and anti-fat violence at the same time. So how can we expect a person the world is hellbent on eradicating to find the internal fortitude to love themselves despite this? Many times, we are navigating a world that doesn't even account for our existence, which is also a form of violence as society seeks to disappear those of us who aren't viewed as worthy through a colonial white-supremacist lens. We are reminded of this by the laws that are passed that specifically target certain populations. For example, 2021 set a record for anti-trans bills in the United States, with 198 being created and many slated to pass. The pandemic has also shed a light on who we view as expendable, which is primarily those who are Black, brown, and Indigenous and disabled people and people with chronic conditions. COVID-19 has disproportionately impacted our communities, and the director of the CDC solidified this fact with her ableist remarks about who is primarily dying from this disease.

Promoting self-love especially through this westernized notion of individuality outside and untouched by society is actually harmful and causes us to miss opportunities to connect with and support each other. It also causes marginalized people to further isolate and then

*blame ourselves for not working hard enough to engage
in self-love despite it all. I personally carry loads of an-
cestral trauma in culmination with what I experience
day to day. I need the type of support that invites me to
fall back into my body. Those of us who are part of multiple oppressed groups need the most love from a variety
of external sources. We need to be celebrated and hon-
ored. Those who are in positions of power and privilege
should be doing all they can to help create more spaces
to provide this support, as opposed to placing the onus
on someone who the world doesn't even think should
exist.*

Ilya's experience also demonstrates the importance of
understanding intersectionality. The term "intersectionality," coined by Black feminist, activist, and lawyer Kim-
berlé Crenshaw, by definition refers to "the interconnected
nature of social categories such as race, class, and gender
as they apply to a given individual or group, regarded as
creating overlapping and interdependent systems of discrimination or disadvantage."

Intersectionality helps us understand that our
identities—how our gender, race, class, sexuality, ability
status, and nationality, among other factors—affect our
lived experiences and the way the world engages with us.
Intersectionality echoes the lessons taught to us by Audre Lorde: "There is no such thing as a single-issue struggle because we do not live single-issue lives." The more

overlapping identities you have, the greater the potential for discrimination, disadvantage, and harm. The important factor to consider about intersectionality is that the overlapping identities are ones that may lead to *discrimination or disadvantage*. For example, being a white woman is not an overlapping identity, as whiteness isn't an identity that leads to discrimination or disadvantage in the world. So for Ilya, it's not just about being Black or trans or nonbinary or fat. It's about all those identities overlapping and creating a very specific experience in the world. One that most of us, myself included, can't truly understand.

In a world that centers thinness, living in a fat body is challenging in ways that those in smaller bodies never think of. Weight discrimination shows up in a myriad of ways, from the size of seating on airplanes and restaurants, to the characterization of fat people in TV sitcoms and movies, to treatment in medical settings. Weight stigma—defined as negative attitudes, beliefs, judgments, stereotypes, and discriminatory acts aimed at individuals simply because of their weight, and specifically aimed at folks in larger bodies—and anti-fat bias are realities that have actual consequences. Here a few of them:

LOSS OF INCOME: Back in 2004, a landmark study found that a sixty-five-pound increase in a woman's weight is associated with a 9 percent drop in earnings. This discrimination basically amounted to losing three years of experience in the workplace. And within the United States, only one state (Michigan) has laws prohibiting workplace discrimination based on weight.

MEDICAL BIAS: A review of studies published in the journal *Obesity Reviews* in 2017 surveying empirical evidence across multiple disciplines showed that healthcare professionals' negative feelings about fat bodies can lead to misdiagnoses and late or "missed" diagnoses, negatively impacting patient outcomes.

CLOTHING BIAS: Many retailers don't sell larger sizes in stores, preventing larger-bodied individuals from being able to easily walk into stores and find clothes that fit their bodies. Plus, there are hella brands (especially high fashion) that don't make their clothes in sizes over 12. And even if clothes are accessible in larger sizes, individuals are often subject to a "fat tax," the difference in price between clothing made for those in the plus-size community (typically beginning at size 14) and clothing that is not. Note that the "fat tax" also applies to things like airplane seats and even bicycles and furniture.

EMOTIONAL DISTRESS: The consequences of weight stigma and having people make assumptions about your health simply because of the size of your body also have psychological impacts. According to the National Association of Eating Disorders, weight stigma poses a significant threat to psychological and physical health. It has been documented as a significant risk factor for depression, body dissatisfaction, and low self-esteem. Those who experience weight-based stigmatization also

- Engage in more frequent binge eating

- Are at an increased risk for eating disorder symptoms

- Are more likely to have a diagnosis for binge eating disorder

WITHIN A RACIST, PATRIARCHAL CULTURE, REMEMBERING THAT the size of our bodies isn't an indicator of our health, our happiness, or our success is often easier said than done, even for the most successful and influential people. Growing up, I remember my brothers and the neighborhood boys being praised with compliments such as "Look how strong you are," while my female friends and I were showered with praise such as "Look how pretty you are." From a young age, I was conditioned to believe that being pretty was the reason for my existence, while boys around me were taught to be strong, athletic, and, of course, brave. Unfortunately, this belief system has followed us into adulthood in many ways. For far too long, society has been overshadowing women's success and accomplishments by making the conversation about women's bodies and their looks, a reality that men are rarely forced to experience.

While there are an endless number of examples of women to demonstrate this phenomenon, two are always top of mind for me: Serena Williams and Adele.

Adele has been blessing us with her angelic voice since her debut album, *19* (named after the age she was when she began recording the project), was released in early 2008. Since then she's gone on to win countless awards, including fifteen Grammys as of 2021. And while her music has always been celebrated, her body, which has had the type of weight ups and downs that are normal and part of life's journey, has been under public scrutiny since the beginning as well. Speaking of this in a 2021 British *Vogue* article, Adele said, "People have been talking about my body for 12 years. They used to talk about it before I lost weight."

In May 2020, Adele posted a birthday picture on Instagram with the following caption:

Thank you for the birthday love. I hope you're all staying safe and sane during this crazy time. I'd like to thank all of our first responders and essential workers who are keeping us safe while risking their lives! You are truly our angels ♥

2020 okay bye thanks x

Although the post only discussed being thankful for the birthday wishes and thanking first responders, the internet went wild and homed in on one thing: Adele had a noticeably slimmer physique. And just like that, the headlines celebrating her new body hit the internet.

ADELE SHOWS OFF IMPRESSIVE WEIGHT LOSS IN STUNNING BIRTHDAY SNAP

ADELE "MAY TOUR AGAIN" AFTER DRAMATICALLY LOSING 45 KG OF WEIGHT

ADELE HIGHLIGHTS WEIGHT LOSS IN STUNNING DRESS AS SHE CELEBRATES 32ND BIRTHDAY IN SELF-ISOLATION

ADELE'S 100LB WEIGHT LOSS RUMOURED TO BE FROM MAINLY PLANT-BASED DIET

ADELE WEIGHT LOSS: EXPERT REVEALS DIET SECRET BEHIND CHISELED LOOKS AND GLOWING SKIN

Adele didn't show up on the internet that day to discuss her body or weight loss, but it was all the internet could talk about for days, with the conversation ranging from praise and celebrations of her weight loss to think pieces expressing disappointment that she lost weight, because for a lot of women in larger bodies, her body and success, in some shape or form, made them feel more comfortable about their own bodies. And when we consider that we don't see a lot of women in larger bodies in the entertainment industry, that perspective does make sense.

In another *Vogue* interview, Adele stated, "My body's been objectified my entire career. It's not just now." Speaking of her weight loss, she added, "I understand why it's a shock. I understand why some women especially were hurt. Visually I represented a lot of women. But I'm still the same person. The most brutal conversations were being had by other women about my body. I was very fucking disappointed with that. That hurt my feelings."

When I read these interviews, I couldn't help thinking that after all the Grammy wins—all the incredible music that she's contributed to the world—the conversation is still about her body. The same body that has been publicly criticized since she was nineteen years old. The same body that was picked apart because she was too large. And now she's having to apologize for letting people down with her weight loss—for what she chose to do with her own body. Not to mention that no matter what she does, her weight and body also seem to take precedence over the conversation, instead of the focus being on her talent and music. Men simply don't deal with this in the same way women do.

The reality is that no matter what Adele or any woman in the public eye chooses to do with their body, people will have something to say. Some will say they liked her better in a bigger body. Others will love her "new and improved" body. People will always and forever have something to say until we get across a really important message to mainstream culture: *It's never okay to give unsolicited comments on anyone's body.* And that is also important for us to reflect on personally. When someone makes disparaging comments about our body or makes suggestions about what is best for our "health" in their eyes, let us remember that if folks are out here criticizing Adele—someone they don't even know personally—they most certainly will speak on our bodies and health. And while it's never okay, it's important for us to remember that the thing that matters most is how we feel about ourselves, because folks are always going to have their opinions.

At the intersection of both racism and sexism, few women have had their accomplishments overshadowed by discussion about their bodies more than Serena Williams has. Arguably the greatest tennis player of all time, Serena has had her career and achievements tainted by incessant rhetoric about her body. From her being called the N-word at tournaments to the constant hypersexuality of her physique, Williams's body has been under persistent scrutiny when really it's her skill as a tennis player that should be the talk of the town. And for good reason. Williams has won twenty-three singles Grand Slam titles (thirty-nine major titles overall) and four Olympic gold medals, spent 319 weeks as world number one, and holds a number of World Tennis Association records. She also holds the most combined Grand Slam titles in singles, doubles, and mixed doubles among active players. The woman is a badass. Period.

And yet, mofos really want to harp on her body. Deep sigh.

But it's beyond just harping on her body. The scrutiny is intertwined with overt racism. Here are just a few of the tweets and comments that have been made about Williams over the years:

Today a giant gorilla escaped the zoo and won the women's title at Wimbledon ... oh that was Serena Williams? My mistake.

Serena Williams is a gorilla.

Earlier this week I said that all female tennis players were good looking. I was clearly mistaken: The Gorilla aka Serena Williams.

My god Serena Williams is ugly! She's built like a silver backed gorilla.

I didn't know apes were allowed in women's tennis.

Yes, I realize the internet is a cruel place filled with trolls and their Twitter fingers, but unfortunately Williams has faced this type of blatant racism at the hands of mainstream media too. In a 2013 article for *Rolling Stone*, Stephen Rodrick compared Williams to a fellow tennis player stating, "Sharapova is tall, white and blond, and, because of that, makes more money in endorsements than Serena, who is black, beautiful and built like one of those monster trucks that crushes Volkswagens at sports arenas."

In 2001, Sid Rosenberg, a prominent sportscaster, said that Serena and her sister Venus would be better off posing for *National Geographic* magazine than for *Playboy*, defending his comments as not racist but "just zoological."

The way in which people have been fascinated with the size and shape of her body more than the breadth of her tennis skills goes back to the intersection of identity at which Black women reside—sexism and racism. Without her consent, Williams's body has been put on display and discussed as if it's an object that doesn't belong to her. As I pored over countless commentaries picking apart Williams's body—the size of her breasts and especially her butt—I was reminded of the legacy of Saartjie Baartman (whom I talk about more in the next chapter).

It's also a perfect time to circle back to that term we discussed earlier, "intersectionality," overlapping and intersecting discrimination. While both Adele and Serena have faced enormous scrutiny from the public, Serena has had to face body shame laced with blatant racism. It's never just about her body—anti-Blackness always rears its ugly head too. Diet culture, fatphobia, and racism go hand in hand, as they are all products of white supremacy.

In juxtaposition, do we ever hear commentary about the shape of Michael Jordan's body? Was his career a constant barrage of critique about being too big or too muscular? No. We simply hear stats upholding why he is the undeniable GOAT (greatest of all time). And he is the GOAT. Granted, I'm no basketball expert (or tennis expert), but have you ever seen those videos of Mike literally flying through the air to dunk? I mean, just watch the 1988 dunk contest. I didn't know such feats were humanly possible. I was sold after that. He's the best. And his career gets to be spoken of as such. He deserves that. But so do women. Women deserve to have their accomplishments just be their accomplishments.

WHAT MUST IT FEEL LIKE TO BE AS POWERFUL, SUCCESSFUL, AND legendary as Serena Williams yet still be judged in this way? There are no easy answers; even the powerful tool of self-love, which is so important, is not the answer to ending our war with our bodies. Self-love as an anecdote to body shame makes it an individual problem. It necessitates that we as individuals are responsible for the way we feel about our bodies and also responsible for our inability to love our bodies with ease. We need to understand that white supremacy, anti-Blackness, and racism are the reasons we struggle with our bodies and face discrimination in the world, and that they are systemic problems, ones that require collective dismantling.

Diet culture and anti-Blackness are at the root of our disdain for our bodies, and promoting self-love as the solution is like treating the symptoms of an infection but never prescribing anything to resolve the infection. Self-love alleviates the symptoms but not the underlying condition. It's a Band-Aid to stop the bleeding. If we don't address the root cause, we will spend a lifetime addressing the symptoms, and the onus is entirely on us as individuals.

White supremacy causes harm to all of us, regardless of identity. However, it's unequivocally more challenging to love yourself when the very essence of who you are is challenged daily. When your body is under attack from every direction, loving yourself, despite all that, is an act of self-preservation. It's vital that we understand that the more intersecting identities a person has, the more difficult radical self-love is. So when we dole out self-love advice that is simplistic in nature, without taking these things into account, we potentially alienate a large segment of the population that perhaps doesn't feel seen or understood. If folks don't have the ability to feel safe in their bodies, no amount of self-love is going to change that.

When I think back to that Target incident, it didn't matter that I knew how smart I was or that I had big plans for my life. It didn't matter how much I did or didn't love myself at that point in time. This man was making assumptions about my intellect and the trajectory of my life because I reside in a Black body, and he held biases and stereotypes about Black people. As a Black woman, I face oppression, discrimination, and marginalization in the world, and no amount of self-love is going to protect or save me from those experiences.

Self-love couldn't save George Floyd, Sandra Bland, Philando Castile, Alton Sterling, Tamir Rice, Tanisha Anderson, Eric Garner, Dontre Hamilton, Korryn Gaines, Breonna Taylor, and countless others from being murdered as a result of police brutality.

So yes, we are more than our bodies, but the implications of the ways our bodies express themselves, and the discrimination that is faced as a result, are a truth we can't escape or sidestep. Our message of self-love is ineffective if we ignore the reality of systemic body oppression, if we fail to address the white supremacy and anti-Blackness at the root of diet culture. That requires that we also address our own racism and anti-Blackness in our hearts and lives.

From Principle to Practice

1. While self-love is a necessary goal for which all of us are deserving, what are your reflections after reading this chapter?

2. How has self-love, although wonderful, not protected you from experiencing harm in the world?

3. How can you work to change some of the systemic barriers and work toward collective liberation for *all* bodies?

4. Have you promoted the message of self-love while ignoring the reality of systemic body oppression (intentionally or unintentionally)?

5. Despite the fact that self-love isn't the antidote to body oppression, how are you working to cultivate a deeper and more loving relationship with yourself?

CHAPTER 3

Decolonizing Our Thoughts about Our Bodies

NONE OF US CAME OUT OF THE WOMB HATING OUR BODIES, CRI-
tiquing ourselves, or obsessively attempting to shrink our
voices. We learned that along the way. That feeling of
never-quite-right-enough is taught to us. It's intentional. It
teaches us to believe that we are never enough. It teaches
us that our happiness lies on the other side of fat loss. It
teaches us to seek perfectionism. It leaves us mired in guilt
and shame when we feel like we don't live up to standards
that we didn't even create.

As it pertains to body dissatisfaction, most of our
discontent stems from ideas and considerations beyond
ourselves. Over the years, we began to adjust and alter ourselves to fit in with the "ideal" standards. It didn't happen
overnight for most of us. It happened little by little, thought

by thought, small adjustment by small adjustment, judgment by judgment, until one day we woke up and we didn't even know how we came to have so much dislike and disdain for ourselves.

We started shrinking and contorting and fixing. We mostly didn't notice it was happening. We often did this in the name of our "preferences" without realizing how our preferences are rooted in white supremacy. But in total transparency, it was likely for the comfort of fitting in or for validation from others, subconscious or not.

Until one day we were no longer able to look in the mirror and like anything about ourselves because we no longer knew what we wanted to be. We only knew what we thought we *should* be. And so, I think the work is to begin unraveling that learned behavior, piece by piece, bit by bit. It doesn't happen overnight. We didn't arrive at this place of dissatisfaction overnight, so we can't expect to return to our true selves overnight.

We do it slowly, little by little, thought by thought, until we come back home to ourselves. Home to the place where we know in our hearts we are enough. We have always been enough. Coming back home to ourselves is the process of decolonizing our minds. Decolonizing our minds means that we deconstruct the thoughts, preferences, and values that derive from a colonial way of thinking.

It was at Calvary Baptist School, the private school I mentioned earlier in the book, that I realized how different I was. Prior to attending this school, I never really thought about my Blackness as being different. I didn't think about my hair as being different. I never felt the urge to prove myself. But there, where most of my peers didn't have any Black friends or neighbors, I was different. It's similar to the Toni Morrison quote, "No one ever talks about the moment you found that you were white. Or the moment you found out you were black. That's a profound revelation. The minute you find that out, something happens. You have to renegotiate everything." This school was where I had a revelation about my Blackness. It's where I started negotiating everything.

I quickly fell into the trap of thinking that I had to be better at everything so that no one would question my worth. We didn't talk about the implications of race much in my household, so I don't know where this line of thinking came from at such a young age. But what I do know is that I quickly decided that I needed to show my classmates that even though I wasn't white, I was just as smart as them. And to be honest, I was smart as hell and regularly scored at the top of my class on tests. I mean, sure there were only twenty kids in my entire class, with the whole school having roughly only two hundred fifty kids, but that's not the point. I was still smart as hell, okay.

Here's the part where I tell you about the second sleepover that I remember vividly. For the sake of this story, we are going to refer to my friend as Julia; that's not the person's real name. The real name is super identifiable, and there's no need to embarrass someone twenty-five years later. I'm chilling at Julia's house, having dinner with her family. We're eating pizza—my favorite. Everything is all good, and then seemingly out of nowhere, Julia proclaims, "My dad doesn't like Black people, but he says you're okay." Y'all, Julia's dad turned beet red and exclaimed, "Julia!" I remember he didn't say anything else. It was like shouting her name was his way of saying that she had said something she shouldn't have said out loud. I wanted to literally disappear at that moment. I just wanted to evaporate into thin air. I was so embarrassed, and I also felt shame. In hindsight, the only person who had a reason to be ashamed was Julia's dad, because he was racist as hell, but I was only ten years old, and this was the first time in my life that I was confronted with the fact that someone might not like me just because of the color of my skin. It was also my first introduction to the idea that certain Black people might be deemed "okay."

Something else happened to me that day. In that moment, I decided that I would do everything I could to be palatable. That's the moment I really adopted respectability politics, "a set of beliefs holding that conformity to prescribed mainstream standards of appearance and behavior will protect a person who is part of a marginalized group, especially a Black person, from prejudices and systemic injustices"—although I didn't have the verbiage at the time. I strove for perfectionism in my life. Perfect grades. Perfect speech. Perfect body. In elementary school, I used to cry if I got a B on a test, and it wasn't because I was going to get in trouble. My parents were fine with Bs. I cried because I was disappointed in myself. Receiving a B was okay, but it wasn't the best. It wasn't perfect.

This carried into other areas of my life well into my late twenties. I contorted myself to be what I believed would be most accepted by the people I interacted with. This influenced the way I talked, the way I dressed, the way I wore my hair, and, most importantly, the way my body looked. I never told anyone about the incident at my friend's house, but it created a narrative that took me nearly two decades to unlearn. If I could go back and talk to my younger self, I would reassure her that the only person who needed to be embarrassed was my friend's dad. I would tell her that her being Black is amazing, even when people like my friend's dad try to make her feel otherwise. I would tell her not to let the world beat her down. I would tell her to fight as hard as she can to resist that feeling of never-quite-right-enough that society will try to impose on her. I would tell her that this is the first of many experiences in life when people will try to convince her that something is wrong with her.

This is my story, but the truth is, we all have these stories. Your story may not be about race or ethnicity. Maybe it's about your sexuality or gender. Maybe it's about mental health. Maybe it's about a learning disability. The details differ but the crux is the same. We are thrust into a world that quickly tells us we aren't enough, and we compare ourselves with others and quickly work to contort ourselves into more acceptable, more palatable versions of ourselves. Versions we think the world will value and appreciate.

For a lot of us, dare I say the majority of us, that involves our bodies, and the lessons we begin receiving at a very early age. According to a recent Dove campaign, 92 percent of teen girls would like to change something about the way they look, with body weight ranking the highest. If I had been asked that question as a teenager, body weight would have been near the top of the list. As I already noted, dieting was heavy on my mind at the age of thirteen.

If you've spent any amount of time doing any of the things below, then you are in good company.

- Comparing your body to other women's bodies

- Looking in the mirror and pointing out your "flaws"

- Feeling frustrated by what you think you "should" look like versus how you actually look

- Feeling like you would be more admired or appreciated if you were thinner

- Feeling like your life would be better or you would be happier if you just lost weight

- Feeling uncomfortable, unworthy, or unpretty in your body

- Hanging on to clothes that no longer fit because you're determined to be that size again

- Buying "goal" clothes as motivation for weight loss

- Worrying about what other people might be saying or thinking about your body

- Feeling incapable of loving or appreciating your body

I have spent more time doing all the above than I care to think about. But how do we all end up in the same place? How do we all find ourselves in negative relationships with our bodies, particularly at such a young age? It's no coincidence that it plagues every one of us, and try as we might, few are immune to the harmful realities of growing up in a patriarchal society rooted in white supremacy. Add capitalism to the mix, and it becomes pretty clear that very few of us have a chance of escaping body image issues or questioning our enoughness. And for those of us with more marginalized identities, it's a double whammy.

The message that we get over and over from the world is that the way we look is the most important thing about us and that we should spend our time, energy, and resources striving for perfection as it pertains to our bodies and our looks. Some of these messages are easy to pick up on, but many of them are much more subtle and subconscious. Jean Kilbourne, a writer who is recognized for her groundbreaking work on the image of women in advertising and her documentary *Killing Us Softly*, spoke in an address given at the Harvard T.H. Chan School of Public Health of the subconscious messages we receive in body-image-related advertisements and how they can create a "toxic cultural environment" that has the potential to harm our relationship with ourselves. An article on Kilbourne's talk summed up her words as follows:

> *The average American encounters 3,000 advertisements every day, and spends a total of two years watching TV commercials in their lifetime, Kilbourne said. At the center of many of these ads is an image of idealized female beauty. Models are tall, slim, and light skinned, and digitally altered to ever-more unrealistic proportions.*
>
> *"Women and girls compare themselves to these images every day," Kilbourne said. "And failure to live up to them is inevitable because they are based on a flawlessness that doesn't exist." The American ideal of beauty has become so pervasive that 50% of three- to six-year-old girls worry about their weight. And on the island of Fiji, the arrival of television heralded a boom in dieting*

among women and girls who before then hadn't realized that there was something wrong with them.

THE BEAUTY AND DIET INDUSTRIES ARE INVESTED IN TELLING US that we aren't enough and that *we need something outside of ourselves to be worthy and deserving of love.* The more they can convince us of this, the more we continue to spend our hard-earned money on the "solutions." The weight-loss market alone is now valued at a whopping $72 billion, and that number doesn't begin to tap into the beauty or fashion industries. Setting standards of beauty that are just out of reach for most of us is a tool of oppression. The late Ayesha K. Faines, founder of Women Love Power, described this phenomenon well.

Standards of beauty are used as weapons against women, and no woman is immune. We tell women that when they get older, you're not valuable anymore. We tell women when they are supposed to look a certain way. We tell women to take up less space. This is the body that's in. No, "this" is the body that's in. We define beauty by such narrow ideals and the intent is to divest women of power, because you become so preoccupied with chasing this notion, and so preoccupied with self-hatred that you forsake the power to go out into the world and be who you were meant to be.

The standards of beauty sold to us are always moving targets. How often do we see blogs or magazine covers with headlines like "Get a J.Lo Booty" or "5 Moves to Get Michelle Obama's Sculpted Arms." Constant reminders of what we should be striving for this month. Next week or next year may be different though.

If we look throughout history, the "in" body is always changing. Standards of beauty aren't static and they never will be. In the 1950s, in the era of Marilyn Monroe, the curvy, hourglass, voluptuous shape was all the rave. By the 1960s, things swung back in the other direction, and thin was back in. Within a decade, women went from striving to be voluptuous and curvy to aspiring to a thin shape, complete with slimmer hips. In the 1980s and '90s, it was the age of the supermodel, so being tall and leggy was the most desirable. Think Naomi Campbell. Fast-forward to the 2010s and onward, and the name of the game is booty-licious. Think Nicki Minaj, J.Lo, and Kim Kardashian.

So desirable is the latest "in" body type that women go to great lengths to achieve that look, safe or not. According to the American Society of Plastic Surgeons, the Brazilian butt lift (BBL), the procedure associated with getting a bigger backside, has the highest rate of death of all aesthetic procedures. However, many of the deaths can be attributed to unqualified practitioners doing the procedure in makeshift surgeries in homes, garages, or motel rooms. So basically, folks are so hungry to have the latest "in" body that they are willing to risk their lives if they don't have the financial means to go to a qualified practitioner. In my opinion, this also goes back to the impact that media, especially social media, has on us all—Instagram in particular. With Photoshop and filters, everyone can look "perfect." I myself have most definitely looked at the body of someone with a BBL and thought, "Wow, I can buy that body?!" Now, I'm not personally going to buy a new body, but that doesn't mean I haven't thought about what I would look like with a bodacious ass. But if I'm being honest, the good Lord knew not to bless me with a giant Georgia peach, because I wouldn't know how to act. I probably wouldn't even have written this book. I would most likely be living in Florida, gainfully employed as someone's sugar baby.

That being said, this is not the part of the book where I shame or condemn plastic surgery. That part of the book doesn't exist. I will never shame anyone for the choices and decisions they make for their own body. That's not my job, and neither is it yours. I believe in body autonomy, the right to make decisions over one's own body. My motto for myself is "My body. My business." However, I do think we should curiously and compassionately interrogate our choices as they pertain to our bodies, because we know that our ideas about bodies and what they should look like have been heavily influenced by cultural standards of beauty and white supremacy. So how many decisions are we even really making on our own if we aren't actively working to decolonize our minds, let alone our bodies?

Speaking of BBLs and the desire for a round Georgia peach, actor Tina Fey states the following in her book, *Bossypants*:

But I think the first real change in women's body image came when J.Lo turned it butt-style. That was the first time that having a large-scale situation in the back was part of mainstream American beauty. Girls wanted butts now. Men were free to admit that they had always enjoyed them. And then, what felt like moments later, boom—Beyoncé brought the leg meat. A back porch and thick muscular legs were now widely admired. And from that day forward, women embraced their diversity and realized that all shapes and sizes are beautiful. Ah ha ha. No. I'm totally messing with you. All Beyoncé and J.Lo have done is add to the laundry list of attributes women must have to qualify as beautiful. Now every girl is expected to have:

- *Caucasian blue eyes*
- *full Spanish lips*
- *a classic button nose*
- *hairless Asian skin with a California tan*
- *a Jamaican dance hall ass*
- *long Swedish legs*
- *small Japanese feet*
- *the abs of a lesbian gym owner*
- *the hips of a nine-year-old boy*

- *the arms of Michelle Obama*
- *and doll tits*

The person closest to actually achieving this look is Kim Kardashian, who, as we know, was made by Russian scientists to sabotage our athletes.

We all know that the Kim Kardashian physique is artificial. We realize that it's an unrealistic expectation for the majority of women to strive for, but that doesn't stop people from going through potentially dangerous measures to achieve it. This leads us to another complicated and nuanced reality. Many BIPOC, Black women in particular, who grew up with naturally larger backsides and naturally big lips, features that now get praised on the likes of the Kardashian crew, were not praised or celebrated for their own features. In fact, it was often quite the opposite. Black girls were berated and teased for exactly those attributes, but now that dominant culture has deemed them "good" and "in style," the tides have magically changed.

This is a perfect example of the myriad of ways in which anti-Blackness is intertwined with body politics. Features that have been traditionally attributed to Black bodies are celebrated and embraced only when someone who is non-Black appropriates and embodies them, even when they are artificial. This is one of the many reasons that for individuals with multiple, intersecting identities, self-love can be that much more challenging.

Regardless of our identity, the beauty industry wants us to believe we can in fact be "perfect." We are just one diet, one beauty product, one haircut away from reaching "perfection." But the reality is that it's a trap. There will always be just one more thing. When I was stuck in my cycle of yo-yo dieting and fat loss, I would reach my goal weight and say, "Just five more pounds." That's what's so insidious about all of this. It's an ever-moving target. We will never be satisfied, and they know that. That's the trap of perfectionism as well. The lie is to believe that we can actually attain the "perfect" body and that once we do, all our problems will be solved. The sun will shine brighter. The birds will chirp louder. We'll find the partner of our dreams. We'll be successful and rich. We'll get the job of our dreams. We'll have more meaningful relationships. We'll be the envy of everyone around us. All because we have the perfect body.

And that's exactly what it is—a lie. I can tell you this from personal experience. In 2014, I was the leanest I had *ever* been in my adult life. I was also in the best physical shape I had ever been in as well. I was deadlifting over four hundred pounds and squatting over three hundred pounds. Those are the things I said I wanted when I got into fitness. I wanted to be "skinny," and then I wanted to get strong. I had accomplished both. But I was miserable, in every sense of the word. Everything that I hoped I would achieve on the other side of fat loss wasn't there. I wasn't happier or more confident in my skin. In fact, I constantly found more things I needed to "fix." I found more "areas of concern." It was a never-ending cycle.

Companies in the diet industry do not, nor have they ever, had our best interests in mind. They aren't concerned about our health. They are concerned with one thing and one thing only: their bottom line. They know that diets don't work. The statistics are available to prove this. But the fact that we keep trying to reach unattainable standards created by them works in their favor. They trick us into believing that the problem lies within. We aren't disciplined enough. We haven't purchased the right exercise plan. We haven't found the right way of eating for our bodies. We keep spending more money looking for the plan that's gonna help us conquer our weight loss once and for all, and they keep getting rich at our expense.

The lie of diet culture is that fat loss is the answer. However, the reality is that on a quest for the "perfect" body, we sink deeper into despair and grow continuously more unhappy with ourselves. In the quest to fix ourselves and find the solutions to man-made problems, we are often left with more body image issues that we started with. It leaves us with complicated relationships with food and exercise. It leaves us with less ability to trust our intuition and trust our bodies. It leaves us seeking perfection again and again and again.

Our obsessions with changing and contorting our bodies are deeply entrenched in a desire to avoid judgment and shame from society. And for good reason. All the depictions of what it means to be "beautiful" shown to us through the media have greatly contributed to our developing implicit biases about our own bodies and the bodies of other people. Implicit bias, also known as unconscious bias, most simply stated is when we aren't conscious of the stereotypes and assumptions we keep. Unfortunately, we have all been conditioned to have ideas about which bodies are "acceptable."

Just think of the portrayal of people in larger bodies on television and in movies. It's commonplace and accepted for fat people to be the object of jokes and poor treatment. It's a form of humor referred to as "fattertainment." For example, the TV show *The Biggest Loser* is devoted to watching fat people perform excruciating hours of exercise and follow dogmatic and restrictive diets with the end goal of losing as much weight as possible. The show coalesces with individuals donning their "new and improved" bodies. The contestants are celebrated for being in smaller bodies.

According to a study entitled "Portrayals of Overweight and Obese Individuals on Commercial Television," published in the *American Journal of Public Health*, media has a huge influence on our implicit bias as it pertains to bodies.

Of 1018 major television characters, 14% of females and 24% of males were overweight or obese, less than half their percentages in the general population. Overweight and obese females were less likely to be considered attractive, to interact with romantic partners, or to display physical affection. Overweight and obese males were less likely to interact with romantic part-ners and friends or to talk about dating and were more likely to be shown eating.

Additionally, the study found that "negative stereo-types are attached to obese individuals, who are often thought to be undisciplined, dishonest, sloppy, ugly, so-cially unattractive, sexually unskilled, and less likely to do productive work, among other attributes. The result is bias and discrimination aimed at overweight persons in im-portant areas of living, including education, employment, and medical care."

All that to say, we are constantly bombarded with mes-sages that have formed our opinions about our own bodies and the bodies of others. We have conflated the idea of what it means to be healthy with a physical look, and we stigmatize fat bodies. We have also put the idea of health and being healthy on a pedestal and use it as a basis of morality. Understanding this reality is what will allow us to see the insidious nature of diet culture and hopefully begin the process of actively decolonizing our minds and seeking liberation for ourselves.

WE ALL HAVE IMPLICIT BIASES ABOUT BODIES, AND FOR A LARGE majority of the population, thinness equates to health. We make assumptions about people based on what their bodies look like. We judge our own worth and how good we feel about ourselves based on the way we look and how "healthy" we are. Also, many of us believe that we have ultimate control over our health. We believe that if we eat well, exercise, and make good choices for ourselves, that we will never be sick, disabled, or chronically ill. When we believe this, we fail to realize that health is a privilege, and it's also quite possible that we have implicit bias around the idea of health in general. When we think of health as a personal choice, it's easy to make judgments about those we don't view as healthy, because it's easy to fall into the line of thinking that they just didn't take good care of themselves or make good choices. But really, that's just our bias showing. There are societal, economic, and social implications that impact health and the choices that we as individuals have access to. Beyond that, when we believe that we have ultimate control over our health, we ignore the reality of life—that we have very little control over anything, including our health. While I absolutely make decisions that support my personal health and well-being as an act of love and self-care, I don't pretend that it will protect me from experiencing sickness or chronic illness. Nor do I believe my health is a factor to be used when it comes to body respect. We all deserve to be treated with dignity and respect, regardless of our health status.

As discussed previously, the body positivity space has been inundated with thinner and medium-sized white women grappling with the ability to love and accept their bodies within an oppressive society that hypersexualizes women and assigns us social status based on our physical appearance. But that raises the question: If women who are more closely aligned with Eurocentric standards of beauty are struggling to accept their bodies, what does that mean for those of us with more marginalized identities? As we understand the implication of race and white supremacy at a deeper level, we begin to recognize that we can't even imagine the difficulty for members of marginalized communities who are attempting to survive and thrive in an inherently anti-Black, heterosexual society. The challenges span beyond just body size, also combating messages about gender, race, ethnicity, sexuality, and ability status, among others.

Fatphobia hurts all of us. This is why when we prioritize dismantling white supremacy and anti-Blackness, first in our lives and then at a systemic level, it provides liberation for all of us. When we focus on body liberation for the most marginalized among us, the result is everyone's liberation. Dismantling and decolonizing are never through the guise of *helping* people with less privilege than we have. They're with the mindset that we are all working toward our own collective liberation. There is no better quote that exemplifies this point than these words often attributed to Lilla Watson: "If you have come here to help me you are wasting your time, but if you have come because your liberation is bound up with mine, then let us work together."

The work is to unlearn our own implicit bias and narratives about bodies, in all their iterations. What are the biases I hold about fat bodies? What are the biases I hold about Black and brown bodies? What are our biases I hold about trans or nonbinary bodies? What are the biases I hold about disabled bodies? These are the questions we have to honestly ask ourselves. It is only through identifying and unlearning our biases and narratives about bodies that we can really begin our journey to body liberation.

RACISM AND WHITE SUPREMACY SHOW UP IN TOXIC FITNESS AND diet culture in a myriad of ways beyond just the racist origins of fatphobia. If you scroll all the way back on my Instagram page, you will see that I used to post "before and after" pictures, something I am now vehemently opposed to. It doesn't matter how you try to spin it: If before and after pictures feature a larger and then a smaller body, we are reinforcing the narrative that smaller bodies are more desirable, more healthy, more preferable. When coaches and trainers post before and after photos of their clients or of themselves, it's meant as a marketing tool to garner more clients—to prove that they can also help you achieve an ideal body. The last time I posted a before and after picture of myself was in 2017 when I was marketing a powerlifting program I created called #PowerConditioning. For the record, that program is top tier and will help you get really strong. I stand behind that 100 percent. But I was still using diet culture and fatphobia to sell the program, with part of the caption reading, "Powerlifting allowed me to change my physique, get leaner, and add some nice curves. Not to mention, I got REALLY STRONG in the process. I lost a ton of inches, changed my body composition, and reduced my body fat." I could have just marketed it as a strength program, but I actively decided to market to people's insecurities by talking about reducing body fat and losing inches while adding curves. That was active participation in toxic fitness culture and diet culture. I was guilty AF. I knew that fat loss sells. It's problematic as hell, but it works, and that's why it continues to be as prevalent as it is. That and the fact that the vast majority of mainstream fitness is fatphobic. They do believe that being in a smaller body is what we should be striving for. I have never taken my old posts down, because as we actively unlearn white supremacy in our lives and decide to no longer be complicit within the system, we pivot, course-correct, and do better. That is the work. But we also don't erase the past. I don't pretend to be perfect. I have absolutely gotten it wrong so many times and still get it wrong sometimes.

For practitioners of wellness, once we realize the interconnected nature of diet culture and racism, we must be willing to actually cut ties with diet culture. When I made the decision to stop coaching people toward intentional fat loss, that potentially meant losing access to capital. Fat loss is the low-hanging fruit. It's the easy way to get more clients, sell more programs, and build your audience by showcasing before and after photos. However, when we operate in this way, we are selling folks the dream that they will feel better about themselves in a smaller body.

This is where the rubber hits the road. Is your commitment to dismantling white supremacy and systems of oppression bigger than your love affair with capitalism? Are people more important than profit? The work of dismantling doesn't occur without personal sacrifice. Again, the reason the beauty and diet industries are committed to convincing us we need to change something about ourselves is for the sole purpose of profit. The more they can convince us of this, the more we fork over our hard-earned dollars for the "solutions." You can't denounce the harmful nature and the way in which it is prohibitive of body liberation while still participating in the system.

Doing this work also means being willing to examine all the ways that white supremacy shows up in toxic fitness culture. Remember earlier we talked about Kim Kardashian and the commodification of Black bodies? How about all the white women selling booty-building programs without acknowledging their ability to profit off traditionally Black attributes that weren't widely accepted until non-Black people tried on these attributes like costumes? The commodification of butts is a form of cultural appropriation, and not only that—it's connected to a racist history as well.

For centuries Black women have been hypersexualized and denigrated because of their bodies. Most notable is Saartjie Baartman, referred to as the "Hottentot Venus." Saartjie Baartman, due to her large buttocks, was paraded around Europe and put on display in freak shows. Her body was literally put on display for objectification. Even following her death, parts of her body were displayed in a Paris museum to support racist theories about people of African ancestry. In a piece for the *Guardian*, Yomi Adegoke speaks of this phenomenon:

> *The era of the big booty has neither started nor ever stopped for black women, and even if it had it wouldn't be the likes of Iggy Azalea, Miley Cyrus or even J Lo we'd be attributing a rear renaissance to. Despite what the mainstream media told us, black women never stopped aspiring to possess the curves society so hated; we chortled in cinemas at Queen Latifah's glee from a yes response to the age-old question "Does my butt look big in this?" in the 2005 comedy Beauty Shop. It was an in-joke; funny, because in a world where white is right, that was most definitely the wrong answer. Yet now, brands puff behind us as they desperately try to catch up, tippex in hand, ready to white up things that have always existed among the minorities they have continually chosen to ignore.*

The commodification of Black bodies is both infuriating and devastating for those of us who live in Black bodies. For many of us who grew up being told our bodies were inadequate to now see those attributes being celebrated on non-Black bodies is a constant reminder of the ever-present anti-Blackness within society.

These are the considerations we have to think about

critically. It is utterly important that we begin to evaluate perspectives outside our own. The question I always ask myself is this:

"If this is difficult for me as a straight-size, cisgender, heterosexual Black woman, what must the experience be for those with additional intersecting identities?" This is a practice we can all embody in our daily lives.

I invite you to take some time to consider your own intersecting identities and dare you to reconcile what life is like for individuals with even more intersecting identities than your own. Facing that reality—that the experience of others may be gravely different than ours—can be a hard truth, particularly if we haven't taken the time previously to consider this perspective.

When I worked with clients on exercise and fitness, I remember distinctly when I decided to stop making fat loss a part of my practice. I personally couldn't, in good conscience, help women pursue intentional fat loss. I wanted to help my clients focus on how they wanted to feel in their bodies—feel stronger, move better, have more energy, etc. If fat loss happened as a result of their movement practice, then so be it. But no longer did I want to help people focus on fat loss as a measure of their "success." When I personally met my fat-loss and weight-loss goals, I did not feel energized, nourished, or whole. I felt anxious, self-conscious, stressed about eating and exercise, and still *not enough*. But more than that, intentional fat loss is diet culture and it is fatphobia. The desire to be in a thinner body is a desire to not be fat. Regardless of the reason, the belief that being in a thinner body is somehow more desirable or healthy than being in a larger body is anti-fat bias. "Fatphobia" is "defined as a pathological fear of fatness," and a lot of folks are simply terrified of living in a larger body. In a 2006 study, almost 50 percent of Americans said they would be willing to give up a year of their life to avoid being fat, and 15 percent reported that they would be willing to give up ten or more years of life. That's how pervasive fatphobia is within our society.

Here are a few more stats:

- In a survey, 75 percent of American women endorsed unhealthy thoughts, feelings, or behaviors related to food or their bodies.

- In 2011, the "obesity industry" (commercial weight-loss programs, weight-loss drug manufacturers, and bariatric surgery centers) was set to top $315 billion, nearly 3 percent of the overall US economy.

- Of "occasional dieters," 35 percent progress into pathological dieting (disordered eating), and as many as 25 percent advance to full-blown eating disorders.

- Weight cycling, or the constant losing and gaining of weight, a result of dieting, leads to adverse health outcomes including a higher risk of death.

If we don't actively work on mindset and recognize our own biases about bodies, we will spend the rest of our lives feeling less than. We have to decide to release beliefs that were actually never ours to begin with. The thing about decolonizing our minds about bodies is that we have to continuously work on it. Colonized thinking shows a preference or desirability for whiteness and cultural values, behaviors, and physical appearances that are derived from western culture—i.e., white supremacist culture. When we are speaking of decolonizing our minds about our bodies, it's also about deconstructing the binary ways of thinking—attractive/unattractive, desirable/undesirable. But even when we recognize that the ideals we have about our bodies and the bodies of others aren't our own—that they're a result of deep programming—we still have to continuously unlearn the harmful narratives we've been taught.

Often body image and self-love are discussed like a destination we get to one day. We finally arrive and now we no longer have negative thoughts about our bodies. Now every single day we wake up feeling awesome in our bodies. However, that's simply not how it works, and I don't know a single person, myself included, who doesn't still have bad-body-image days. We all do, and we can't expect ourselves to never have those days. The days occur less frequently for me now than they used to, but they still show up. The goal is not to ignore those feelings or will them away. The goal is to sit compassionately with those feelings as they arise and to acknowledge that it's really challenging living in a world that makes us feel like there's something wrong with our bodies. It's hard living in a world that makes us think we are supposed to have a flat stomach, no wrinkles, no cellulite, no rolls, a small waist, a big ass, no hip dips, lean and toned arms, and on and on and on. It's difficult. A colleague of mine, Jenna Jozefowski, once stated that working on your relationship with your body image is like brushing your teeth. You do it every day. Hopefully. I really hope y'all are brushing your teeth every day.

But the point is, we don't just brush our teeth once and never do it again. It's a daily practice, and for me, so is working on my relationship with myself and my body. It's a relationship that requires care and attention. You will have bad-body-image days. You will see your fatphobia creep back up. You may have days when you compare your body with someone else's. I'm sorry I can't tell you that body liberation makes those things disappear into the abyss forever, but I can say that it allows for the occurrences to appear less frequently and allows you to flip the narrative much quicker.

Decolonizing our minds is a necessary step in the journey toward liberation, and yet, let us always remember that it's like peeling back the layers of the onion. We keep questioning the thoughts that pop into our minds and the ways in which we are intentionally or unintentionally participating in diet culture. Fatphobia is deeply ingrained in our brains and society as a whole, and we have to continuously unlearn it in our lives. Not only for ourselves but for the liberation of everyone. So that hopefully future generations don't have to go through all the bullshit we do. So that hopefully one day we stop sitting in those feelings of not-quite-right-enough. In the words of Hollie Holden:

Today I asked my body what she needed.
. . .
She whispered, very gently:

Could you just love me like this?

From Principle to Practice

1. Take a moment to write down your own intersecting identities.

2. How have your identities impacted your experience in the world?

3. What privileges do you have as a result of your identities?

4. Consider what dismantling diet culture in your life, and collectively, may require of you.

5. For the next week, jot down on your phone each time you hear someone mention a colonizing statement about bodies—whether it be in passing on the street, on TV, in a film, in a conversation with your family, in advertising, etc.

CHAPTER 4

Breaking Up with Diet Culture and Examining Your Privilege:
What It's Costing You and Others

IN 2019, I DECIDED TO GO ON A TRIP TO SPAIN WITH A GROUP OF Black women I didn't know. I was invited by Monique Melton, whom I had met only once prior to the trip. Monique is an anti-racism educator, podcaster, and author. We met because she attended a retreat hosted by me and two of my friends earlier in 2019. Monique is someone I now consider a good friend, but at the time, I barely knew her, if I'm being honest. Some people might think that sounds bananas, but I'm a Sagittarius. I rarely say no to a trip or the prospect of a good time. I spent a week in Madrid with a group of women, who would end up becoming friends, and I did what would have felt impossible just a few years earlier. I devoured chocolate croissants, delicious cakes, and every other pastry that tickled my fancy. I feasted on paella, beef cheeks, delectable hams, and cheeses and enjoyed Spanish tortilla. And I quenched my thirst with more glasses of wine and sangria than I can count. The most amazing part of it all? I didn't spend even one minute of time feeling any shame about how much I consumed. There were no quips about how "vacation calories don't count" or how I'd have to "go extra hard in the gym" to make up for all the food I ate on my trip—none of that occurred this time around. I never felt bad about what I would have previously considered "overindulging." I was so fully present and enjoying the memories being created. It was pure bliss. It felt like freedom. Freedom to really experience life and not be obsessing about my body or weight gain.

If I'd taken this trip even five or six years earlier, things would have been drastically different. My relationship with food was much more complicated back then. I was deeply entrenched in diet culture and obsessed with maintaining a smaller body at all costs. I tracked every morsel of food that entered my mouth and weighed myself daily, and just the thought of going on vacation and not having total control over *exactly* what I was consuming gave me extreme anxiety. That felt like the opposite of freedom. I felt like I was trapped. The irony is that at that time, I was tracking my macros, which is also called "flexible dieting" because you can supposedly eat whatever you want without depriving your body of specific foods, but I felt anything but free. Eat whatever you want as long as it fits into your macros. It's totally flexible—not a diet at all.

In hindsight, of course, it was absolutely a diet. It's literally called flexible dieting. Quick sidebar: This is the part where people get really upset. How dare I call flexible eating or intuitive eating—or whatever trendy name it has nowadays—"dieting." This is also the part where you may feel compelled to write me an email about your personal success story of finding more balance through this approach or how it actually helped you eat more or how you feel better when you track. Please save it. Do not email me, DM me, @ me on Twitter, or send me a carrier pigeon. I said what I said. The word "diet" is in the name, and I spent years of my life on this diet while simultaneously claiming I wasn't on a diet. I could eat anything I wanted—Pop-Tarts, cake, candy, anything—as long as I didn't go over my macros. Duh . . . not a diet at all. I had truly convinced myself that I was just being "healthy," and I was a real smug bitch about it too. Like I really thought my discipline made me morally better than other people. I assured myself that I cared more about my health than everyone else did, but at the same time, I was also miserable because I hated it when I wanted to eat something that didn't fit in my macros. I would either acquiesce and eat it anyway and subsequently wallow in guilt and shame, or I wouldn't allow myself to have it and make some low-calorie bullshit version of it.

This period of my life is the reason why, to this day, I

get angry when I see a cauliflower or zucchini version of something. Like, I don't care how y'all market it, pureed cauliflower does not taste like mashed potatoes. Zucchini noodles, also called zoodles, don't taste like pasta. THEY JUST DON'T. On food-prep Sundays, a term that actually makes me sick to my stomach now because I would spend at least four or five hours of my life each Sunday in order to ensure I was prepared to stick to my macros, I used to make these sweet-potato protein muffins. Y'all, the ingredients included xylitol sweetener (a sugar substitute), vanilla protein powder, and get this . . . sweet-potato baby food . . . BABY FOOD. They tasted like the tears of disappointment, but I convinced myself that they were delicious and ate them for months on end. I kid you not, I actually get nauseous when I think about them now. In fact, we need to move on. I can't talk about it anymore.

But the point is, my life felt really small and constricted at that time. My family knew that I wouldn't do anything that would conflict with my workout schedule, and if I was in a situation where going out to eat was involved, I would eat as little as possible during the day so that I could "splurge" at dinner. During my corporate-job years, I would take sick leave for doctor appointments during the day but really just go do a workout if I couldn't make it to the gym after work for some reason. And for the record, I feel zero remorse about that. When I quit that job, I had over four hundred hours of sick leave for which I couldn't get paid. In hindsight, I probably should have taken more sick leave.

When I was in college on one of my many yo-yo diets and I wanted to go out on the weekends, there was a period when I would eat only egg whites and a slice of toast twice during the day so that I could use my calories for alcohol. Do you know how quickly you get drunk off vodka and Diet Coke when you've barely eaten real food all day? Very drunk, very quickly. The things I did in the name of keeping my body small. Those were all disordered eating behaviors, by the way.

Diet culture has in many ways robbed us of the experience of food. It's led a lot of us to forget that eating can and should be a pleasurable experience, not one riddled by fear of gaining weight. I'm sure we've all heard the phrase "food is fuel." Yes, that's true, but food is also so much more than just fuel. When we think of food only as fuel, it discounts so much of the essence of food. Food is an experience. Food is culture. Food is memories. Food is pleasure. Food is a way to share love with one another. When we make food an issue of morality, labeling food as "good" or "bad," or "healthy" or "unhealthy," not only do we rob ourselves of the pleasure of eating, but it leads us into a cycle of guilt and shame about eating, an act required to live. And also, our ideas of what foods are good or bad are deeply embedded in racism, white supremacy, and fatphobia.

The foods we classify as "junk food" or "calorie dense" or "hyperpalatable" (for the folks who want to act like they're not demonizing food, even though they are—diet culture is a tricky little bitch) are usually items high in calories and sugar, and we deem them "bad" simply because eating a lot of them could lead to weight gain. And yes, folks will argue that it's also because they aren't very nutrient dense, but really it always comes back to people's fear of gaining weight. It's also about the way diet culture praises foods like kale while demonizing people's cultural foods, especially foods associated with BIPOC cultures, like rice, biscuits, pasta, and tortillas. Foods that are more culturally aligned with whiteness have historically been upheld as the "right" way to eat, especially if it's a salad with "all the colors of the rainbow" present. And is there anything that makes a white lady happier than eating a salad? Seriously. Just pause here and google "woman eating salad" and you are going to be assaulted by an ungodly amount of overzealous white women eating salads. Who knew greens could make one so happy?

I would be remiss if I didn't at least mention the issue of food apartheid (often referred to as "food deserts") and accessibility when we are talking about food as well. The push for "organic" and whole foods is steeped in racism, ableism, and capitalism, as it doesn't account for the fact that large portions of the population simply don't have geographic access to quality fresh fruits and vegetables or the means to feed their entire families grass-fed, non-GMO, unprocessed, "fed only the best," "allowed to run around in the sun," pesticide-free—and whatever other things I'm missing—meat. I am a single (fairly privileged) woman, and I can't get out of Trader Joe's without spending at least $100, so I can't even fathom what it costs to feed an entire family. When I was growing up, there were lots of times our family food budget was tight, not that my parents necessarily talked about it, but it was obvious. We ate cheap meals that easily fed all of us, things like pots of spaghetti or Hamburger Helper with a side of canned corn or green beans. Perhaps it wasn't the most "nutrient dense" or fresh food, and for damn sure not organic, but it allowed us to survive. You can decide for yourself which one is more important.

But more than just robbing us of the experience of food, diet culture robs us of the beautiful experience of life. How much time and energy have we spent worrying about how we look or feeling so uncomfortable in our own skin that we are unable to be fully present in each moment?

When I was the absolute smallest that I ever was as an adult, I have so many memories of being so self-conscious in my body that I spent entire outings at the beach or the waterpark obsessing about how I looked and sucking in my stomach as hard as I could. I remember accomplishing big milestones during periods when I had regained weight and being excited but wishing that I were skinnier because somehow that would have made the success just a little bit better. At the time, I felt like that would have allowed me to be proud of my accomplishments *and* proud of the way I looked.

Here's what I didn't understand at the time, and again, what I've learned through body liberation: *Our bodies are simply the vessels that allow us to have this human experience.* They don't make us who we are. At our core, we are not our bodies. Our bodies are just the shell we reside in.

I've said this before, but it bears repeating. Body liberation isn't about looking in the mirror and loving everything you. It's about understanding that in our essence, we are more than our bodies. Stephanie Chinn, illustrator, artist, and author of *Here Sister, Let Me Help You Up*, whom I became acquainted with through Instagram, put my thoughts into perfect words, stating, "This body is just the keeper of my magic." That's exactly it. This body, this shell, is simply the container that houses all the incredible magic that is in every single one of us. We've all been sold the lie that the way our body *looks* is the magic, but that couldn't be further from the truth.

The more we identify as our bodies, the more we struggle to find peace within ourselves. The truth is, this body is fleeting. It could all change in an instant. The way it looks, the way it moves, the way it feels—that's all going to change. In fact, our bodies were designed to do just that. The sooner we internalize and accept this, the easier body liberation becomes. You can feel free to love your body in all its iterations because you know that it will go through countless iterations from birth to death.

When I lost a bunch of weight during my junior year of

high school, I had to buy some new clothes to accommodate my smaller body. I remember splurging (for a teenager's budget—remember I was making those big Target bucks) and heading to Express. I bought a few pairs of jeans, but I had a favorite pair that I will never forget. They were the perfect mix of new and already worn-looking. They were fairly straight-legged, had the perfect-sized hole in the left knee, were just the right color—not too light or too dark—and had a washed-out pattern across the front. They might not sound like much, but, y'all, these jeans were legit. I loved these jeans so much, but what I think was my favorite part is that they were a size 8. I do not remember ever wearing a size 8. I always joke that I came out of the womb an adult size. I don't have any recollection of shopping in the kids' section as a child. I vividly remember shopping in the adult section in third and fourth grade. For the record, it's hard to look like a child when you have to wear the same clothes as grown women. Plus, my mom never took me to cool places to shop. She used to take me shopping at this store called the Dressbarn. The Dressbarn! I have no idea if that store is still around, and if it is, and you like it, please don't be offended. But at ten years old, it just wasn't cool.

So anyway, when I bought these jeans, I felt like I had finally achieved what I had always wanted. I was finally in a small body. But the problem was, I had achieved my "goal body" by super unhealthy and unsustainable methods. So as yo-yo dieting tends to go, I would inevitably gain some weight back and the jeans wouldn't fit anymore. But in my mind, the jeans represented my ideal size, so I always held on to them, even into my midtwenties. There would be periods when I couldn't fit into them, but they were always there, waiting for me to shrink back into them. When I comfortably fit back into them, I was temporarily happy again. And each time, I would promise myself that this would be the last time I would have to fit back into them. This would be the time that I would be able to sustain the weight loss. I wasn't going to fail at another diet.

But of course that wasn't true. Statistics estimate that about 95 percent of dieters regain everything they lose and then some within three years. This is also one of the reasons the diet and weight-loss industry is a $72 billion industry. If diets worked, would people be continuously spending copious amounts of money trying to achieve their dream bodies? Diets don't work, but the promise of finding the "perfect" plan keeps people motivated to try the next best thing in hopes that this time it will be the thing that works for them. And the diet industry has realized that people are starting to wise up to its predatory tactics, so it has gotten trickier in its marketing. For example, Noom is an app that claims it's not a diet and instead promises to help you "Change how you think. Change how you eat. Change for good," while simultaneously prescribing members low-calorie intakes and encouraging people to track everything they eat for optimal success. It's not a diet, but it casually mentions on its website that 78 percent of Noom users lost weight over the course of a six-month study. Intentionally eating in a manner aimed to reduce body fat is a diet. Period.

I don't think people fail at diets. I think that diets and diet culture have failed us. According to a 2020 poll of two thousand participants, the average person will try 126 fad diets over the course of their lifetime. The poll also found that the average person will embark on two fad diets a year, which will typically last less than a week. Over half the participants admitted to being really confused about which diets were sustainable, with a large number also stating they didn't know where to get reliable or truthful information about diets and weight loss. The most disturbing part of the poll is that one in twenty people stated that they would be happy to intentionally ingest a tapeworm to burn calories.

Diet culture has led us to believe that all bodies are supposed to look the same—thin. It's really interesting, because every day we look at people around us and see genetic differences that we never question. Some people are tall, while others are short. Some of us have brown eyes, while others have blue or green eyes. Hair colors vary from brown and black to blond and red. We are all blessed with different hues. And yet we question none of this. But when it comes to bodies, we can't accept that bodies are also meant to look different. We aren't all supposed to be thin. We aren't all genetically predisposed to live in a small body.

Every one of us could eat the same thing and do the exact same exercise program and we would all look very different. Regardless of how much we diet, restrict, or exercise in an attempt to keep our bodies small, some of us just weren't meant to be skinny.

Fatphobia and racism have somehow made this idea, that all bodies are created to be thin, the dominant thought process. And we have bought in and indoctrinated it into our society as almost fact or truth, even though we know it's not. For example, the body mass index (BMI) is bullshit, and at this point, it's fairly common knowledge. First, it was developed by a man named Adolphe Quetelet, who, believe it or not, wasn't even a medical professional. He was an astronomer and mathematician, besides being a eugenicist. Red flag number 1. Second, Quetelet developed the equation using height and weight data from only white European men, most of them middle or upper class, so it wasn't at all representative of the general population. Another huge red flag. Finally, it's completely arbitrary and not a good indicator of health. Despite all that, it's still used to determine things like health insurance premiums and disability insurance premiums, as well as your risk for certain conditions such as diabetes and heart disease. Also, doctors may use this number to inaccurately assume that all health ailments are related to BMI and easily could be eradicated by reducing it.

Since BMI was developed on the basis of data from white European men, it doesn't account for gender, race, or body composition and therefore disproportionately impacts women and BIPOC. I mean, this seems like an obvious "Duh," but of course my body doesn't measure the same as a European white man's body. I'm not really into labels, because they're subjective, and plus they change like the wind, but I'm a fairly straight-size Black woman. I typically wear a size 12 in clothes. In a multitude of ways, I benefit from thin privilege even though I don't consider myself a thin woman. I can go into stores and find clothes that fit me. People rarely comment on my food choices or question my physical capabilities when I enter a gym space. I don't have to deal with a lot of shit that people in larger bodies have to deal with, and yet, according to the BMI chart, I am obese with a BMI of 34.02. I know that because I recently had to have a bunch of blood work done in addition to being weighed because I was applying for disability insurance. I don't give a rat's ass about being labeled "obese." The reality is that I think the word is problematic and harmful for a lot of reasons, including the stigma and judgments that are associated with it. In addition, it unfairly penalizes people for basic human rights—another form of the fat tax—for falling into an arbitrarily created category. For the record, all my test results were fabulous. I'm not exaggerating—actually fabulous. My cholesterol is so great that my doctor was even impressed, but because I am obese by BMI standards, I will pay more for insurance. To be clear, my belief is that no matter how much someone weighs or what their blood work looks like, everyone deserves access to healthcare and insurance, and none of us should have to pay more. It's a basic fucking human right. My point in telling you this story is to illustrate that the BMI is bullshit, and it is not an indicator of our "health." Just as the sizes of our bodies are not an indicator of our health.

But one of the reasons that so many of us pursue fat loss, whether we realize it or not, is that we want access to the privileges that come with living in a smaller body. Thin privilege represents all the social, financial, and practical benefits a person gets because they are thin or in a relatively smaller body. The world accommodates and centers thin bodies. Even if you don't consider yourself a thin person, the closer you are to Eurocentric standards of beauty, the more you benefit from thin privilege.

I grew up extremely sheltered. My mother loves Jesus with her whole heart. I often joke that she has Jesus on the mainline, and when I'm struggling with something, I ask her to pray for me because, as I tell her, "God hears all your prayers as a priority. You're VIP." There were a LOT of things my siblings and I couldn't watch on television growing up, ranging from *Power Rangers* to *Sabrina the Teenage Witch*, and definitely no Disney movies. To this day, I have still never seen an episode of *The Simpsons*. I've also never been trick-or-treating, but that's another story for another day.

Sometimes I would sneak and watch shows I wasn't supposed to. One of those shows was *Baywatch*. I remember the first time I saw Pamela Anderson running down the beach in that infamous red one-piece. She was skinny, had legs for days, and had huge breasts. A few days after I first laid eyes on Pamela Anderson on *Baywatch*, I remember being at the grocery store and seeing her on the cover of a magazine, being touted as one of the most beautiful women in the world and described as a blond, busty bombshell. A blond, busty bombshell?! That sounded amazing. Who wouldn't want to be described as a bombshell and lauded as the most beautiful woman in the world?!

This was the '90s, and if you think mainstream industries lack representation now, just imagine how dire the representation was back then. These were the images I was being inundated with as beautiful—long, flowing blond hair and blue eyes and Barbie-doll bodies. How was a Black girl with kinky, curly hair supposed to be able to achieve Pamela Anderson–like beauty? I could never achieve long, flowing blond hair or blue eyes or white skin, but I could try to be thin. I could try to achieve a beautiful-looking body, and maybe the world would see me as beautiful too. Being in a thinner body was a desire for proximity to whiteness and privilege. As a little girl, I obviously didn't know that, and I have so much compassion for her and the many versions of her that existed over the years.

I spent a lot of time chasing thinness. But what I finally realized as an adult is that no matter how much I changed and contorted myself, I would never be able to attain Eurocentric standards of beauty, which are rooted in white supremacy and racism. While grasping for access to privilege at the expense of my body, I was also battling my own internalized anti-Blackness and fatphobia. It wasn't about my health, because the things I put my body through weren't healthy. I wanted to be skinny, and hopefully that would also include being healthy, but I don't think I really cared about the health part that much at the time. If someone would have asked me back then if I would have eaten the same way and exercised the same way if it didn't result in weight loss, the answer would have been a resounding "Hell no." In fact, I can't even count the amount of times I lamented the fact that I wasn't one of those people who could eat whatever they wanted and not gain weight. I referred to those people as "lucky." So many of the things we say about "health" are really just our own fatphobia and biases.

One day I had an epiphany. I realized that my favorite jeans from high school weren't supposed to fit my grown-ass woman body anymore, so why did I keep retraumatizing my body to shrink back into them? I say "retraumatizing" because every yo-yo diet I did, which always involved restriction and overexercise, caused trauma to my body. How ludicrous would it be to expect my sixteen-year-old body to fit into the clothes I wore when I was six? But at some point, I decided that my high school body was the one I was supposed to hang on to for the rest of my life. When I finally let go of those legendary Express jeans, I felt free.

Free from ever expecting my body to fit back into them. I was finally able to allow my body to take whatever form it wanted, while showing it all the love and care it deserves.

And if you can still wear your high school jeans, that's cool too. The only point I'm making here is that bodies change, and it's normal. They were created and designed to do that. They change shape and size. They age. They deteriorate. They wrinkle and dimple. They lose hair and grow hair in new places. They lose weight. They gain weight. They deal with chronic illness and disease. Some of them birth children. Some of them run marathons. Some of them use wheelchairs. Some of them have fewer extremities. Some of them have more. There is an endless amount of ways to have a body, and there is no right or wrong way to have one. That is the beauty of our shared humanity.

All our bodies carry us through so many experiences, and no matter how much we try to hang on to the illusion of control, so much of life truly is unpredictable. For example, COVID-19. Did I ever imagine that a virus that primarily enters the body through the eyes, nose, and mouth and progresses into the lungs, causing potentially serious illness and even death, was going to inflict the entire world, and we would be forced to stay in our homes for long periods of time and wear masks when we went outside? Did I imagine that I would be so paranoid and terrified that I would clean the packaging of my groceries with Lysol disinfecting wipes as soon as I brought them home? Did I know that I would grow so anxious about germs that

I would start washing my hands like I was scrubbing in for surgery (this is not a joke—just ask my best friend, okay)? Of course I didn't know. That sounds like some futuristic movie, not real life. But it happened, and if I learned nothing else from living through a pandemic, it's just how fleeting and unpredictable our existence is. No matter how much you plan and try to control, so many things will simply not go according to your plans.

Speaking of bodies changing, my body certainly looks different than it did pre-COVID. My thighs are thicker. My waistline has undoubtedly gained a couple inches. My body is softer where it was once more defined. When I think about my own body and how it's changed over the past few years, I'm reminded that this is a body that got me through some immensely challenging and traumatic times. I don't consider my body perfect, and perhaps you don't either. But I stopped asking my body for perfection a long time ago. My body does so much for me, and I refuse to be convinced that it's not worthy or needs fixing or needs to "get back in shape" or back to the way it looked pre-COVID. Instead, I wake up every single morning grateful that I'm still here in this vessel experiencing life, regardless of how I may feel about my body on that particular day.

The truth is, this body is fleeting. It could all change in an instant. The way it looks, the way it moves, the way it feels—that's all going to change. We can't predict when or how these changes are going to occur. And no matter how much we exercise or how "healthy" we eat, we don't have ultimate control over what happens. What happens if we put all our value in our bodies and our external appearance and suddenly we feel as if our bodies have failed us because of a chronic illness or natural aging, never mind a sudden accident? How will we find the ability to love our bodies if they don't perform in the ways we are used to? What's left then? What's left when everything we thought we were comes crashing down?

It's very likely that the body you reside in today is different from your body from five years ago. It's also very likely that your body five years in the future will be different from your body today. That's okay and normal and part of the human experience. That being said, we work toward loving, respecting, and appreciating our bodies in all of their iterations. And that, my friends, is why we choose body liberation. We choose freedom.

Freedom from obsessive thoughts about changing or manipulating ourselves to fit into societal standards of beauty.

Freedom from obsessive thoughts about every morsel of food you eat.

Freedom from expectations—other people's and our own.

Freedom to disavow diet culture, toxic fitness culture, and systemic oppression that wants to keep us at war with ourselves.

Freedom to feel comfortable in your body in all its iterations.

Freedom to enjoy and savor food and truly be present in our experiences.

Freedom to embrace and actually love the person that you are.

Freedom to always remember that this body we reside in is just a shell that allows us to have a human experience.

Freedom to examine and process our own internalized fatphobia.

Freedom to make decisions about our bodies for ourselves, free of external influences and conditioning.

Freedom to feel bad about whatever we want and remember that we deserve the same grace, self-compassion, and kindness that we show everyone else.

Freedom to reclaim our time and our bodies.

Freedom to unapologetically take up as much space as you want.

Here's the reality: You could spend your entire existence worrying about the way your body looks, and you could allow it to cloud your achievements, taint your accomplishments and celebrations, and dull your experiences. But whether it's a pandemic, a chronic illness, a change in lifestyle, birthing a child, or simply the process of aging, all our bodies will continue to change. They were designed to do that. It's inevitable.

The journey to body liberation is hard at times, but it's one of the most worthwhile endeavors we can ever pursue for ourselves. As we embrace liberation, we are able to celebrate and appreciate the body we have right now—in its current shape, size, and ability level. That's what embracing body liberation has done for me. It's allowed me true freedom in my body in all its iterations. What a tragedy it would be to spend the best moments, days, or a lifetime fighting with your body and wishing it were something else.

I spent so much time and energy obsessing about my body, and it was all a waste, because *the least interesting thing about me is the way I look*. I know it might sound cliché, but it's what I really believe to be true. What I finally realized after a lot of pain and heartache is that I was spending my limited time on earth obsessing about this shell that was designed to change and designed to deteriorate. I was missing out on life and all its beauty because I was trapped in a cycle of body shame and preoccupation.

Although it's not an easy task by any means, we can choose to break up with diet culture and fatphobia and create a reality that is not stifled by food, the scale, or an obsession with our bodies. When I'm on my deathbed, the memories I cultivated along the way are the things I will relish. I won't look back and wish I would have denied myself a decadent slice of cake or maintained six-pack abs at the expense of my sanity and well-being. I will, however, reminisce on the memories I created with people I'll never forget: Picnics in the park with friends. Glasses of wine on the patio keekeeing with my homegirls. Ice cream post-dinner because we are enjoying the company and the laughter so much (and because ice cream is delicious, of course). Weekend getaways to new cities just for the hell of it. I can't think of Spain without remembering the amazing chocolate croissants I ate with my friends Tash and Monique overlooking the beautiful city of Madrid. On my deathbed, I'll reminisce on the experiences this body allowed me to have.

Do you remember back in 2017, when Representative Maxine Waters fought back against a white male cabinet secretary who was trying to straight up waste her time and mansplain to her, and she repeatedly hit him with the phrase "reclaiming my time"? She went on to say, "When you're on my time, I can reclaim it." Auntie Maxine is a straight-up badass. She is not to be played with. I think it's time we channel some of that Auntie Maxine energy as it pertains to diet culture. We have agency over our physical bodies, and even while living in a society that is jacked up as it pertains to bodies, especially women's bodies, we can decide to reclaim our time and our power. Diet culture has been robbing us—of our time, of our joy, of our love for ourselves, and even of our potential. We are reclaiming our time and our lives, to live on our own terms, ones that do not include missing out on the best experiences of our lives because we were wishing our bodies were different.

You could spend your entire existence worried about how your body looks.

You could allow it to cloud every experience that you have.

You could allow it to cloud your achievements.

You could allow it to dull your accomplishments.

You could let it be the thing that taints your celebrations.

You could let it be the thing that always makes you feel just not quite good enough, despite all your success.

Or you could not.

Because life is short.

Our existence is fleeting.

You deserve pleasure and joy now—in your current body.

Not when you lose a few pounds.

Not when you achieve the body of your dreams.

Not when you achieve the ideal hourglass figure.

I want you to know that your looks are the least interesting thing about you. You are whole, complete, and unconditionally loved, and none of that has anything to do with the vessel you reside in. I want you to know that I understand it's hard, but it's worth fighting for liberation. I don't want you to spend your best moments, days, or a lifetime wishing your body were something else. What a tragedy that would be. Refuse to let that be your story.

Spain was the trip when I realized I had truly found body liberation. It's when I knew diet culture and fatphobia were no longer in the driver's seat of my life. I had reclaimed my time, and I was free. I would be lying to you if I pretended that I never find myself tempted to fall prey to

societal standards of beauty. But when I do, I quickly remind myself that attempting to live up to standards that
are ultimately rooted in white supremacy and racism only
keeps me trapped and bound. And I am choosing freedom.
Over and over. Day after day.

This shell that we reside in does not make us who we
are. It simply allows us to have this human experience, and
I hope you choose a reality filled with joy and fullness, free
from self-loathing. We have no idea how long we get to
have this human existence. Life is short. Time is fleeting.
Tomorrow isn't promised. May we not spend our precious
time obsessing about the size of our bodies.

From Principle to Practice

—

1. How have you obsessed about maintaining a thin body?

2. Have you struggled with accepting your body in all its iterations?

3. Since the origins of fatphobia are deeply embedded in white supremacy, how have you, intentionally or unintentionally, upheld diet culture?

4. In what ways are you holding on to previous (thinner, stronger, younger) versions of your body without recognizing that your body is just the vessel you exist in, not who you are?

CHAPTER 5

Acknowledging the Harm You May Be Causing Others, Part 1:
The Inclusivity Band-Aid as a Block to Liberation

THE WORD "PRIVILEGE" TRIGGERS PEOPLE—ESPECIALLY WHEN YOU put the word "white" in front of it. If I had a dollar for every time I heard a white person denounce having privilege by sharing that they, too, struggled with a hard life or grew up poor, I would be a very, very rich woman. I would likely be living in my own private villa on the blue-green waters of Turks and Caicos, complete with a private chef and personal masseur. Okay, maybe that's an exaggeration, but I would definitely be living bicoastal and flying first class everywhere I go.

However, the reality of privilege—which by definition means a special right, advantage, or immunity granted or available only to a particular person or group—is that we all possess privilege of some sort. We have access to privilege based on a myriad of things such as race, gender, education, economic status, ability status, body size, and many, many more. It goes without saying that while we have access to privilege, some of us have more access than others. And if we were to talk about the privilege pyramid (I'm not entirely sure that's even a real thing, but stick with me), cisgender, straight white men are certainly at the top of the pyramid.

As we seek personal liberation from the oppressive throes of diet culture and begin to work on repairing our relationships with our own bodies, we have to begin to question and understand the role of privilege in our own lives. It's important to understand that it doesn't make us bad people. It doesn't mean that we haven't had hard lives or had to struggle. So when we speak of white privilege, it doesn't mean that members of the dominant group grew up with silver spoons in their mouths or had everything handed to them on a platter. In fact, I doubt that's true for the majority of people. But what it does mean is that the color of their skin hasn't made their lives more difficult.

Acknowledging our privilege can feel like a hard pill to swallow, but in order to challenge and dismantle systems of oppression, we have to accept the realities of it. It's difficult to change what we don't accept. Unfortunately, often our privileges are invisible to us until we begin to look at the experiences and treatment of those different from ourselves. While we seek to be anti-racist, it's imperative that we always consider our privilege and how it impacts our experience of the world.

While we often hear discussions about how to "use our privilege" for good, it's important to recognize that the goal of anti-racism is to dismantle the system of white supremacy that allows for privilege, white privilege specifically, to exist. That means disavowing access, entitlement, and the benefits that accompany it. Without the system of white supremacy, white privilege is meaningless and no longer exists. That being said, the goal isn't to "use our privilege for good"; the goal is that white privilege no longer exists.

As I previously mentioned, the events of 2020 following the murder of George Floyd reignited anti-racism discussions among the masses. Everyone was suddenly recommitted to diversity. White people were wallowing in guilt and shame, unaware of how to help, and so the #AmplifyBlackVoices hashtag commenced. I myself, along with many fellow Black creatives, was suddenly being inundated with requests from individuals eager to talk about racism and the need for more inclusion. My name was being spread all over social media in an attempt to "pass the mic." So while the intention may have been good, and it was somewhat encouraging to see people finally wake up to the realities of racism in America, it's normal that I would question the authenticity of this resurgence of anti-racism. Were people really interested in dismantling white supremacy, or were they concerned they would look bad if they didn't say something? And more importantly, how had all these people not realized racism was a thing prior to this point?

And this is where we circle back to the word "privilege," my friends. White privilege allows members of the dominant group to essentially live in their own bubble and not acknowledge the oppression of Black and brown people until a man loses his life and it's spewed all over the internet as Black trauma porn, the media portrayal of racism, Black death, and the ongoing suffering of Black people. I often wonder what was so unique about the murder of George Floyd that it led to global awareness. Was it because we were in the middle of a pandemic and for the most part at home? Was it because of the social media era, and that information is literally at our fingertips and spreads like wildfire? I ask these questions because the reality is that George Floyd wasn't a phenomenon. In fact, he's just one of many individuals needlessly murdered at the hands of the police. Why didn't the murders of Sandra Bland, Philando Castile, Alton Sterling, Tamir Rice, Tanisha Anderson, Eric Garner, Dontre Hamilton, or Korryn Gaines, or the countless other Black people who had their lives taken by the very individuals who are supposed to serve and protect, lead to a global awakening?

For all BIPOC, but especially for Black folks, the murder of George Floyd didn't suddenly wake us up to the realities of racism. We live that reality every single day. And to be honest, as an educator doing the work of anti-racism in wellness, it was kind of a slap in the face to have individuals who had never been interested in being anti-racist suddenly showing up on the internet using their platforms to "amplify Black voices."

WHITE PEOPLE I DIDN'T KNOW WERE SENDING ME MONEY VIA PayPal, Venmo, Cash App, and even via carrier pigeon. The last part is obviously a joke, but the point is, the money was flowing in by any and all means. They didn't know what to do, but goddammit, they were gonna give their money to Black folks, especially those with a social media following. They were going to compensate us for the free labor we were doing on the internet. Slavery was over, goddammit. They were not like their ancestors, and they were gonna pay reparations. They were gonna right the wrongs of all the "bad whites."

I kid you not, there were days during June 2020 when I literally received hundreds of dollars from white people whom I had never met, much less heard of, because George Floyd had been murdered. I'm going to be 100 percent transparent. Although I had no idea how this was going to dismantle white supremacy, I didn't return one red cent, because, I mean, my ancestors were enslaved people. I considered it a redistribution of wealth, if nothing else. I also was physically and emotionally drained, so it paid for the DoorDash and Uber Eats habits I took up during that period of my life. And I was really intentional to order from Black businesses at least 75 percent of the time, so #SupportBlackBusinesses.

I have jokingly said that my next book is going to be a collection of essays entitled *That One Time Racism Almost Made Me Rich and Other Stories*. Maybe it's a joke. Maybe I'm manifesting it. I guess time will tell. But the sad reality is, I made more money during 2020, the year white people suddenly realized racism was still a thing, than I did in any other year of my life up to that point.

And I want to be clear that it's not because I capitalized off the moment and came up with some fancy, new shiny object to sell. I literally kept doing the same exact things I had always been doing, writing about and doing workshops about creating an anti-racist and inclusive wellness industry. People just finally started listening. If you don't believe me, just google me. My work on these topics predates the George Floyd era. I have been discussing the importance of anti-racism and diversity and inclusion in fitness and wellness long before the events of 2020 because the necessity of the conversation has always been there, regardless of whether the masses recognized the importance or not. I'm not new to this, I'm true to this.

It's a difficult and nuanced pill to swallow. On one side of the coin, to finally be fairly and adequately compensated for my work is a good thing. On the other side of the coin, people only cared because a man was murdered on camera, it was internationally televised, and suddenly people *finally* believed that racism was real and something to be concerned about. It's disheartening at best.

I have so many stories to illustrate my frustration with the fitness industry and the reason for my valid skepticism of all the individuals suddenly interested in being anti-racist. A few years ago, after I had begun speaking out about the need to discuss anti-racism and inclusiveness specifically as it pertains to fitness and wellness, I had a little run-in with a well-known fitness influencer and entrepreneur named Megan. At the time, Megan had over half a million followers. I had only a few thousand; however, I was already becoming a leader in the industry when it came to talking about the intersection of racism and fitness. Megan reached out to me to ask for my opinion about how to handle a situation that had occurred online with one of her friends. Her friend was being called out for using the N-word. Both of these women were white, and she wanted some advice about how to handle it. I don't even remember what the conclusion of the conversation was. But what I do remember is that I helped her, out of the goodness of my heart, without financial compensation, although she did send me some free fitness apparel. Have you ever tried to pay for your groceries in free apparel? Let me spare you—it doesn't work. For the record, ya girl is much smarter now and that would not happen today. Slavery is over, and I do not work for white people for free or out of the goodness of my heart.

But anyway, back to the story. Months later, and Megan is being called out for a new apparel line in which she is using the word "savage." One of the many things I have spoken and written about is how important language is, especially when we are seeking to create inclusive environments. I even wrote an article specifically about why the fitness industry should stop using "savage." Back at this point in my journey, I hadn't quite gotten a grasp on my role within liberation work. It was clear that part of my work was speaking truth to power, but I didn't have any boundaries in place yet. That being said, people would DM me about every wrongdoing occurring on the internet, and I thought it was my responsibility to get involved. A few people, several of them Indigenous, reached out to me about the apparel line after expressing their frustration to the influencer responsible for the shirt and not hearing anything back. After hearing about the overall issue and all the anger out there, I felt confident that I could have a productive conversation with this woman. I had helped her with a race-related issue with her friend just a couple months before. Well . . . all I can say is that I was so wrong. After crafting a perfectly compassionate message with all the same level of caution that you would approach a toddler (because let's be honest, we know white women can be fragile), she still chose to respond with fragility, victim blaming, and the worst excuse—she had "checked with some of [her] other friends of color and they said it was fine." Facepalm.

To be honest, I shouldn't have been surprised, but I still was. I wish this was where the story ended, but that would be too easy. In the following days, I started getting messages from other well-known influencers within the fitness space, with large platforms, many of whom I had never spoken with, letting me know that this woman was essentially starting a smear campaign against me, telling everyone I was crazy. I was infuriated, but I also realized that this is just the reality of being a Black educator and content creator, and especially a Black woman. As soon as you don't do exactly what someone wants, you become the angry Black woman, even though you were amazing a few months ago when they needed something. It's the quickness with which whiteness will discard you when you no longer serve their needs. For me, this was just affirmation that the change I was hoping to create within the fitness and wellness industry was absolutely necessary. It was also the moment I realized that if I was going to continue doing this work, I would have to develop tough skin and better boundaries because the world isn't always kind to Black women, especially when they have the audacity to speak truth to power.

Fast-forward to June 2020, when I had decided to relaunch some of my Anti-Racism and Diversity and Inclusion (D&I) courses for fitness and wellness professionals (by the way, these are still available on my website for purchase #ShamelessPlug), and guess who is shouting my praises to the rooftops all across several of her social media platforms and encouraging everyone to sign up for my courses? You guessed it. This same woman. Do you think she ever reached out to me to apologize or address what happened in the past? No. A resounding no. She never acknowledged anything that had happened. But she wanted to make sure the world knew that she was supporting a Black woman, taking my course, and encouraging everyone to do the same. She wanted everyone to know that she was one of the good ones. And this, my friends, is performative allyship, "activism done to increase one's social capital rather than because of one's devotion to a cause," at its finest.

And while we are talking about allyship, can we sidestep for a second to address the elephant in the room? White people reading this do not get to self-proclaim yourselves as allies. By definition, an ally is an individual who speaks out and stands up for a person or group that's targeted and discriminated against. Allies work to end oppression by supporting and advocating for those who are stigmatized, discriminated against, or treated unfairly.

The term "ally" is not a title you can claim for yourself. Being an ally is an action, not an identifier. It's exemplified by the way you live your life. It's fine for members of historically excluded communities to refer to others as allies. But it's not something that you should walk around calling yourself; the statement—"I am an ally"—is in itself performative. Performative allyship is arguably just for show, and awarding yourself the title of an ally does nothing to further the causes of the actual communities you claim to care about.

And besides, instead of trying to be an ally, seek to be a co-conspirator, someone who chooses to take action against racism regardless of the consequences. To be a co-conspirator is about commitment, trust, and love for the cause. It is about relinquishing your privilege in the battle against racism. Allyship is about working to support and advocate for those who are oppressed, while being a co-conspirator is indicative of someone who is willing to risk personal sacrifice to dismantle systems of oppression. And let's be honest, that requires a lot more than allyship.

So much of the conversation following the events of 2020 revolved around diversity and inclusion statements and initiatives. Everyone wanted to slap a Band-Aid on the issues. Inclusion was that Band-Aid. It quickly became a race among companies, influencers, and everyone in between to announce to the world that they were focused on diversity and inclusion because everyone deserves to feel welcome. After leading thousands of individuals virtually through anti-racism and D&I training, I had companies spanning from small yoga studios to the likes of Under Armour reaching out to me for private training. Ninety percent of them were requesting D&I training or something related.

During this period, I realized that a lot of folks want to defer to the importance of diversity and inclusion when the thing we really need to be confronting is white supremacy. Focusing on D&I feels easier than talking about what actual liberation for all of us would mean and require. Inclusion is simply the bandage that stops the bleeding temporarily. For those of us who have suffered the pain of the wounds and trauma caused by racism, the bandage does nothing. The reality is that inclusion, although important, is often a block to actual liberation. There are lots of definitions of the word "inclusion," but the one I like best is by Ferris State University, which defines inclusion as "involvement and collaboration, where the inherent worth and dignity of all people are recognized." It notes that an inclusive organization "promotes and sustains a sense of belonging; it values and practices respect for the talents, beliefs, backgrounds, and ways of living of its members." Too frequently it focuses on making changes to existing practices without recognizing that the systems in place are inherently biased and racist. Dismantling requires just that—breaking down and starting over.

Without being firmly rooted in anti-racism and paired with solid action, diversity and inclusion are just terms that sound good but lack any real meaning.

Inclusion is a block to liberation because many of the same companies, organizations, and individuals reaching out to me to educate on their platforms via podcast, Zoom, and social media were asking me to work for free or in exchange for "exposure." And for those willing to pay, my rates were often out of their budget, and they requested that I accept a lower rate because this work was so "important." This completely misses the mark on inclusion and equity. This is what happens when you focus on looking like you're doing the right thing for outward appearances instead of actually doing the right thing. If your goal is to focus on diversity, inclusion, and equity, but you don't want to pay Black educators for their work, aren't you still operating under the auspices of racism and white supremacy?

For the record, every time I'm asked to do something for "exposure," I want to email back and tell them that it's clear I already have exposure. I mean, after all, that's how they found me, right? I've obviously been exposed enough for them to find me. I trust that I will continue to be discovered without their assistance. I will only accept my payment, especially for the work of anti-racism and D&I, in dollars.

Liberation means freedom in lots of ways, and part of that is pay equity. True equity means that we address the fact that Black women make sixty-three cents to the dollar of white men. So you can't possibly be trying to dismantle white supremacy while simultaneously trying to undercut the pay for the very educator you are bringing in to talk about racism and D&I.

Inclusion is often the roadblock to actual liberation, especially body liberation, because this is the place where the conversation stops. People take the courses and webinars and read the books and believe they have "done the work." But reading is not the work of anti-racism or body liberation. The work of anti-racism is an ongoing action in our daily lives. Understanding and doing the work of anti-racism is absolutely necessary to body liberation because so many of our ideals about our bodies are rooted in white supremacy. Which bodies are deemed acceptable. Which bodies are worthy and deserving of respect and dignity. Which bodies are viewed as beautiful. Which bodies are allowed to feel safe in their skin. As we do the work of anti-racism in our lives, we also decolonize our ideas about our bodies.

When we slap the word "inclusive" on all things body positivity without interrogating what it means to create true inclusivity and without realizing that we really need to be talking about equity, not just inclusion, we block true liberation. With everyone's newly found commitment to inclusion, what we really witnessed is people using members of historically excluded communities as props in the name of inclusivity. This is especially true in the body positivity space. Companies were suddenly creating inclusive campaigns with the sole purpose of . . . showing how inclusive they were. As a leader within the body positivity space, although I don't actually identify my work as such, I was being requested to join every panel regarding diversity and inclusion. But the reality is, true inclusion means that Black creators are being invited to be the experts on all sorts of topics, not just to share their experiences or trauma to convince people about why diversity and inclusion is important. And most importantly, true inclusivity doesn't require that you announce to everyone that you are doing an inclusive event. However, folks often do this because what matters most to them is letting other people know that they are doing the right thing, even if the actions don't truly create an impact.

It's also a well-documented fact that Black influencers continue to be paid less by brands than their white counterparts. According to data from MSL Group, a global public relations firm, the racial pay gap between white and Black influencers is 35 percent, bigger than any other industry on record.

I saw firsthand how many white influencers in the body positivity space took to their Instagram pages starting in June 2020 to let their audiences know they were listening and learning. They shared the posts, posted their black squares, and most definitely amplified the voices of BIPOC. But the problem is, that's not the work. How many of those influencers have actually stood in solidarity with BIPOC creators to end the racial pay gap in the influencer space? How many of those influencers are not only refusing to work on campaigns unless the campaign is inclusive but also demanding that the pay be equitable? How many of those influencers are engaging in pay transparency, which is something that could actually help eliminate the pay disparity?

And this is the reason I say that inclusivity is a

Band-Aid to liberation: because it allows people to believe they are doing their part without actually sacrificing anything. And the reality is, there is no liberation without sacrifice. If members of the dominant group aren't willing to pass up opportunities, money, and even relationships to demand justice and equity (and yes, that includes financial equity) for all bodies, we aren't doing the work of body liberation.

Now, more than two years after these events, we can reflect and see if those newly interested in anti-racism were actually committed to the work or if it was merely performative, as many were worried about. According to a study from Creative Investment Research, US companies pledged $50 billion toward racial equity following Floyd's murder, but since then, only $250 million has been spent on or devoted to a specific initiative. That said, it seems a lot of folks' concerns with performative activism, aka performative allyship, were valid.

Seeking only inclusion is harmful to body liberation and collective liberation because it doesn't actually do the work of dismantling. It allows folks to look good and also feel good about themselves without actual devotion to the cause. When one engages in anti-racism in a performative nature without taking any accountability for past actions or without actually being willing to let go of proximity to privilege, it's harmful, not helpful. Left in the aftermath is everyone who is still being harmed by systems of oppression. While hundreds of thousands of people put up black squares to virtue-signal their solidarity with Black folks, we (Black folks) were left wondering what the tangible actions were.

My friend Monique Melton is the founder of Shine Brighter Together, a community dedicated to pursuing Black liberation through building a daily practice of anti-racism, and she coined the term "pseudo white awakening" to describe these events. Melton states:

Pseudo white awakening is a term I coined to describe what happened following the events of the summer of 2020. What we experienced was a significant increase of white folks pretending to notice something, that thing being racism, that they had the opportunity to ignore for so long. What really ignited the pseudo white awakening was a surge of white guilt, which led to white urgency in very large numbers. You had all these folks acknowledging racism for the first time, even though the reality is that racism has always been occurring. The pseudo white awakening was really just grand performative allyship. You had a lot of folks engaging in behaviors and antics for the sake of appearance. This was due to several reasons. People wanted to appear like they weren't one of "those white people" so it led to an increase of white exceptionalism. Some people did it to be relevant. Then you had people who engaged in order to avoid backlash for not saying anything. All of these reasons are very self-centered and lead to the slippery slope of performative allyship, which ultimately ends in white apathy. Folks are not fulfilling the promises they made and industries have gone back to not discussing racism at all. Folks are dropping off in every aspect of the work because they were never in it for the right reasons. Performative allyship has nothing to do with the people being harmed and everything to do with the person who wants to appear like they are aligned with the folks suffering. If the motive is to alleviate guilt or gain social capital, once that is achieved, there's no need to do anything more. Posting the black squares and the hashtags was enough to achieve what they wanted. They were never truly interested in Black liberation or redistributing power.

While diversity and inclusion can be important, they are not anti-racist in nature. The reality is that liberation takes real work, a commitment to change, and the willingness to cede power. Ceding power often feels like oppression to individuals who are accustomed to privilege and power. The talk of diversity and inclusion is the easy part. The work required is much harder. Often, this is the part people never get to.

The work of anti-racism and dismantling white supremacy, and ultimately liberation, is not work that you pick up and put down as it's convenient for you. Black people don't have the ability to take off their skin to avoid discrimination, anti-Blackness, or oppression when it's too exhausting. The work of creating a wellness and fitness industry that is anti-racist, diverse, inclusive, and equitable isn't business strategy. It's not the type of work you embark on to make your company look good, nor will it be easy or comfortable. It's work that you embark on because you truly desire to create an anti-racist industry and are committed to this mission for the long haul. This work is a marathon, not a sprint.

What the summer of 2020 taught us is that the pseudo white awakening was overwhelmingly self-serving and reactive. As I previously mentioned, after a few weeks, people lost interest, and soon everyone's newsfeed was back to business as "normal," proving, as so many of us feared, that most of the support received was performative in nature.

The work of anti-racism is an ongoing action in our daily lives, and it's 100 percent necessary for the goal of body liberation. Collective body liberation requires that all of us stay committed to dismantling white supremacy and systems of oppression even when it's not convenient.

From Principle to Practice

———

1. In what ways do you hold privilege in your life?

2. How have you been complicit in your life as it pertains to anti-racism and body politics?

3. How have you used Black and brown bodies, along with other historically excluded communities, as props in the name of "inclusivity"?

4. Are you doing anti-racism work in your life, not just in words but in practice? If you are, in what ways? If not, what specific actions are you willing to commit to in this moment?

5. Doing the work of anti-racism in the quest for collective liberation requires we have difficult conversations with those closest to us. Can you commit to "doing the work" by utilizing your voice with those closest to you (family, partners, friends, peers)?

CHAPTER 6

Acknowledging the Harm You May Be Causing Others, Part 2:

The Trauma Loop

EARLIER IN THE BOOK, I SHARED AN EMAIL I RECEIVED FROM A very upset individual for having the audacity to talk about white supremacy. But really, she is the one with the audacity. I actually prefer to call it "caucacity." I don't know who exactly coined this term. It wasn't me, but it's honestly the perfect word to describe some of the scenarios I find myself in, and the best part is that the word has officially made it to Dictionary.com. Let me just tell you—Black folks create culture. We do. It's just that simple. We started casually using the word "caucacity" to describe the audacity of white folks and now it's on Dictionary.com. Wow. We are that amazing. By definition, "caucacity" is a "slang term used to make fun of behaviors perceived to be stereo-typically white or to call out what's seen to be a particu-larly bold instance of white privilege or racism." It's the audacity of white people and their willingness to act in ways that only their white privilege allows them to.

Much of the work I do concerning anti-racism and white supremacy is focused on the wellness industry. There's a reason for that. There's a lot of caucacity happen-ing in the wellness industry. I got into fitness as an enthu-siast and quickly realized the multitude of problems with the fitness space—the racism, the fatphobia, the ableism, the elitism, the homophobia, how much it catered to a thin, white audience, how inaccessible it was, and the list goes on and on. I didn't have a name for it. I just knew what I was seeing. Ilya Parker, founder of Decolonizing Fitness, would years later coin a term for this, "toxic fitness culture." It is defined by them as "social characteristics, language and habits that promote/reinforce ableism, fatphobia, racism, classism, elitism, body shaming/policing, LGBTQIA+ hatred under the guise of fitness and wellness. Toxic fitness cul-ture is rooted in white supremacist ideals regarding health, ability, size, gender, age and beauty. Toxic fitness culture and diet culture are intertwined, with both placing blame on an individual for the ways their body shows up in this world." I love this definition because, yes, what I saw hap-pening was a product of diet culture but also so much more than just that alone.

We just talked about the pseudo white awakening of

2020 and how during that time I relaunched some of my courses. Thousands of folks signed up, y'all. Thousands. The overwhelming majority of them were white people. While I do believe that I had a meaningful impact on some of those participants, sometimes I really wonder if what I'm doing actually effects change or just provides white folks an opportunity to feel better about themselves for "doing the work" without actually doing anything. There's a reason I say this. I have countless examples to demonstrate why I frequently delve into this line of thinking. I tell you these stories because I think it's important to note that it's easy to point to the large, public celebrity fails—when some A-lister uses the N-word or makes a blatantly racist tweet—but the reality is that ordinary, everyday people engage in problematic and racist behavior in the same way, just without the large public audience. In my opinion, these everyday encounters with ordinary people matter just as much, if not more. I encourage you to think about your own behavior, especially as a member of the dominant group. How do you respond when you are called in or called out by a Black person or person of color? Do you unfollow, block, and move on, or do you address it thoughtfully and intentionally? Let me share a few of these stories with you.

First, there's the story of Annie, a white fitness coach with a relatively large following. If this story sounds a little similar to the story in the last chapter, it's because it does bear a lot of similarities. Annie was someone I had been following on Instagram for a while. Her fitness knowledge was legit, and she didn't include a lot of diet culture BS. I had never heard Annie talk about inclusivity, much less even use the word, but days after the tragic murder of George Floyd, she jumped on the bandwagon, posting the words "I can't breathe" as well as the all-important black square showing her solidarity, while simultaneously letting her audience know she was now using her platform to educate and challenge, followed by an explanation of white privilege. To show her commitment, Annie also pointed her audience to myself and other Black educators as "resources" on the topic of anti-racism, also mentioning that she was intentionally adding more Black women and WOC to the mix. That statement was particularly triggering to me because Black women and WOC aren't props you just "add to the mix" when you suddenly decide you need to be more inclusive. And of course, the most important step, she signed up for my course and let everyone know she was taking it.

I'm not sure how long Annie stayed committed to her quest for "inclusivity." I'm not sure what, if anything, she implemented. But fast-forward a few months, and Annie was up to some caucacity. I'll spare you the details, but essentially, she made a post that was not only problematic but actually antithetical to anti-racism. I attempted to have a conversation with Annie, hoping we could have some thoughtful dialogue about the problematic nature of what she posted, and how did Annie respond? By blocking me. She blocked me and refused to even have a conversation about it. By this time, people were also calling her out in the comment section of her post, which she addressed by deleting all the negative comments, leaving the ones that praised her, and eventually disabling the comment section altogether. When confronted by a Black woman, the very woman she had turned to for anti-racist education, Annie responded with fragility and chose to disengage.

Then there's the story of Danielle. Danielle reached out to me because she runs a women's movement collective and wanted me to come speak about diversity, equity, and inclusion (DEI) at one of their events. We had numerous phone conversations, and one of the things we discussed was that she really wanted the event to be inclusive and wanted my input on things, especially if I noticed anything that didn't feel aligned with that mission. I agreed to speak, although there was no compensation, and traveled to the event with high hopes. Throughout the weekend, there were several large misses when it came to the event actually being inclusive. I didn't bring it up at the time, because I didn't want to disrupt the flow of their weekend. However, about a week after the event, I sent Danielle an email expressing some of the highlights of the weekend as well as some concerns and considerations for future events. Danielle, the woman who literally asked me to give them feedback, not only responded with fragility but also ended up blaming some of my feedback on me, as if I were the issue. I replied back to her email, politely expressing how her fragility was showing up and explaining that discomfort is part of the work of anti-racism, and guess what? I never heard from her again.

Finally, there's the story of Debbie. After attending some of my workshops, Debbie reached out for private training for her large fitness franchise. Her company had never addressed issues of race, but following George Floyd's murder, she said she understood the importance and wanted me to do some DEI training for her company. I informed her that I would be willing to work with them only if we started with anti-racism training. She agreed, and in the end she hired me to do a six-part series for her company. Prior to the first training, she reached out and requested a meeting because a decent amount of her franchisees had expressed concern about having anti-racism training, stated that it had nothing to do with fitness. I informed her that people being uncomfortable with anti-racism is par for the course, especially since she had never addressed matters of race before. Debbie said she understood but asked me to be delicate. I informed Debbie that I teach all my courses the same, that I lead with love and compassion, but we talk about the difficult things, and there is no way around that. During the first training, it was obvious there was a lot of frustration among the franchise owners on both sides—the few BIPOC on the call were frustrated and fed up, while the overwhelming majority didn't want to talk about race. After the first training, Debbie said my services weren't needed anymore. While she'd enjoyed my training, her company just wasn't ready yet. She said she would pay me the remaining balance of my contract and we would revisit it in the future. A few days later, one of the white franchisees reached out to me personally to inform me that Debbie had updated the company website to say that they had completed extensive anti-racism and DEI training and that it was one of their company missions. I asked her if she had addressed Debbie, to which she responded that she had not and felt it probably made more sense for me to do so. I didn't bother to address the matter with Debbie, but as you can imagine, I also never heard from Debbie again.

HERE'S THE THING. WHITE PEOPLE LOVE COMFORT. THEY LOVE the ability to show up to anti-racism when it's popular and trendy, but to simultaneously have the ability to fall back when it becomes too cumbersome or uncomfortable or inconvenient for them. They can collect the accolades for "being on the right side" and then go back and serve their own needs when it best suits them. Not to mention, it's a healthy ego boost for them when their white followers show up in their comments to applaud them for their "bravery." Nothing like white folks praising each other for doing the bare minimum as it pertains to racism. I'm not exaggerating about white folks not being fond of discomfort, especially as it pertains to conversations about racism. Recently, Florida governor Ron DeSantis gave first approval to a bill that would prohibit schools and private businesses from making people feel "guilt" or "discomfort" about the country's racist past. Good Lord, not an actual bill to ensure white folks don't have to feel discomfort addressing this country's ongoing racism as well as its racist history! Instead of creating bills that protect and ensure the comfort for everyone living in this country—Black folks, POC, and the 2SLGBTQIA+ community—bills are being created to protect the feelings of those who have historically caused harm and continue to even today. This is white supremacy in action. It's upholding white fragility and giving white people a free pass to ignore their racism.

As a Black woman, I am telling you that it is exhausting, frustrating, and traumatizing. The thing we don't talk about enough is that Black people, Black women in particular, have been out here working toward liberation for a long time. It's not because we necessarily want to save humanity; it's because we want to save ourselves. And when we save ourselves, when we work to dismantle white supremacy, everyone else benefits. Unfortunately, what we continue to experience as a result of advocating for ourselves is also trauma, often at the hands of the very people we have worked with. From slavery to the wage gap to attempting to measure up to Eurocentric standards of beauty, we are also carrying so much intergenerational trauma. In many ways, this trauma has left Black women feeling like we are the lowest class of citizens in the United States. Malcolm X spoke of this in a 1962 speech delivered in LA, stating, "The most disrespected person in America is the Black woman. The most unprotected person in America is the Black woman. The most neglected person in America is the Black woman."

The other thing that we don't talk about enough is that when the Annies or Danielles or Debbies of the world wreak their havoc, we don't see enough of our white peers actively calling this behavior out. If we wish to be co-conspirators, we have to be willing to hold our peers accountable when we see them engaging in problematic behavior. When our peers cause public harm, we must be willing to hold them accountable publicly. Far too often, white women are allowed to cause public harm to BIPOC and marginalized communities with little to no consequences.

This is not a "woe is me" moment. This is a moment to examine how individuals doing the work of anti-racism are continuously experiencing trauma while simultaneously trying to heal from the collective racial trauma. When the wellness industry finally realized racism was a thing in 2020, people were pulling me in all directions because they needed help right now. It was an emergency for them. Their businesses were in a state of crisis as they scrambled to deal with conversations related to racism that they clearly weren't equipped to have. I was being inundated with requests for paid work, but also for unpaid work—podcasts, newsletters, interviews for articles, IG Lives, and everything you can think of.

I wonder if any of these folks stopped to consider the impact that the murder of George Floyd was having on us—Black educators. We were experiencing collective grief, trauma, and anger. We were being subjected to Black trauma porn on every outlet, from the news to Twitter to

Instagram. In an effort to "raise awareness," people were sharing the video of Floyd's murder everywhere without considering the impact this had on the Black community. Our trauma was being exploited, and all the while, Black educators were being tasked with educating white folks about racism.

And then, there's the additional and equally important question of compensation. I saw this coffee mug on Instagram that read, "Pay Black women for their labor instead of using them for diversity clout." I wholeheartedly agree. Before you ask anyone from a historically excluded community to work for free, pause. But especially, if you ever intend to ask a Black woman to educate or speak on matters of racism or diversity, equity, and inclusion for free, it's a full stop. Imagine the irony of asking someone to teach about racism for free, as if slavery isn't a thing of the past. Imagine the irony of asking a Black woman to talk about DEI for free, as if equity doesn't include pay equity. Pay us. But also respect us. Stop referring to BIPOC as "resources." Black women (or any other members of historically excluded communities) are not commodities to be used and tossed aside when it's no longer convenient. It's dehumanizing. I am a full human being who sometimes educates on anti-racism. The reality is that it is not my responsibility or my life's work as a Black woman to educate on anti-racism, white supremacy, or DEI or to be a resource for such topics, especially for free.

But I choose to do this work because I really believe that wellness is for everyone, and I believe everyone deserves to feel welcomed, celebrated, and affirmed within wellness spaces. Wellness isn't about Downward Dogs and green smoothies. It's not just the physical. It's about mental, emotional, and spiritual health as well. All these aspects of wellness have an impact on physical health. In addition, experiencing racism impacts physical health.

In his 2016 TED Talk, David R. Williams, PhD, MPH, a professor at the Harvard T.H. Chan School of Public Health, stated, "America has recently awakened to a steady drumbeat of unarmed Black men being shot by the police. What is even a bigger story is that every seven minutes a Black person dies prematurely in the United States. That is, over two hundred Black people die every single day who would not die if the health of Blacks and whites were equal."

In this talk, he goes on to discuss a myriad of health implications caused by experiencing discrimination and racism, including increased levels of stress hormones, high blood pressure, increased instances of heart disease and breast cancer, and even premature mortality. In addition, Black women are two to three times more likely to die from pregnancy-related causes than white women, and COVID-19 deaths among Black Americans are substantially higher (92.3 deaths per 100,000 people) than among white Americans (45.2 deaths per 100,000 people), according to the Centers for Disease Control and Prevention.

When you think about the impact that racism has on health, it's imperative that BIPOC have access to wellness to combat the negative impact that racism has on both our physical and mental health; but what good is wellness if we enter those spaces and are also subjected to anti-Blackness and racism? Part of liberation is being able to freely navigate the world. This is one of the reasons I choose to do this work within the wellness industry. But unfortunately, it often results in an ongoing trauma loop. BIPOC experience racial trauma; white folks wake up to the realities of racism and are now interested in being less racist; Black educators like me facilitate courses, trainings, workshops, etc., on white supremacy and racism; and finally, completing the loop, white folks cause harm to the very individuals they looked to for education.

THE STORIES I SHARED ABOVE ARE NOT ISOLATED. I CAN TELL YOU story after story of being harmed by the very people who sought out my services for education. Anti-Blackness within wellness culture is par for the course, which is also why so many people have begun intentionally carving out wellness spaces created specifically for Black women, like my friend Les Alfred, creator and host of the podcast *Balanced Black Girl*, which provides content and community, creating safe spaces for millennial Black women to live their healthiest lives. While I love spaces created specifically for and with BIPOC in mind, we also shouldn't have to create those spaces *just* to avoid being harmed.

What does this have to do with body liberation? It has everything to do with body liberation because trauma lives in the body. How can anyone achieve body liberation and feel safe in their body if their nervous system is constantly being disrupted by racial trauma? Instances of racial trauma don't just affect us in the moment; they continue to live with us and generations to come as well—i.e., intergenerational trauma.

> *Traumatized people chronically feel unsafe inside their bodies: The past is alive in the form of gnawing interior discomfort. Their bodies are constantly bombarded by visceral warning signs, and, in an attempt to control these processes, they often become expert at ignoring their gut feelings and in numbing awareness of what is played out inside. They learn to hide from their selves.*
>
> —Bessel A. van der Kolk, *The Body Keeps the Score: Brain, Mind, and Body in the Healing of Trauma*

I don't pretend to be an expert on trauma, but I am an expert on myself, and I've seen the impact of ongoing racial trauma in my life—the fear of being pulled over by the police, chronic fatigue and anxiety following another racialized attack on a person who looks like me, and lately, when it all feels too overwhelming, the inability to acknowledge or even process ongoing racial trauma. Choosing numbness sometimes feels easier.

Far too often and for far too long when conversations are raised about racism, anti-Blackness, and white supremacy within the wellness industry and the trauma they cause, the response is that we need to focus more on "love and light." Toxic wellness culture also loves to lean into toxic positivity, an obsession with positive thinking and the belief that people should put a positive spin on all experiences, even those that are profoundly tragic. The "love and light" crowd, aka the spiritual-bypassing crowd, runs rampant in the wellness industry.

Rachel Cargle, writer, social entrepreneur, and founder of the Loveland Foundation, wrote the following:

> *The easiest way for white women to skirt around the realities of racism is to just "love and light it away." When confronted with the ways they have offended a marginalized group with their words or actions, they immediately start to demand unity and peace; painting those they harmed as aggressive, mean, or divisive. I don't want your love and light if it doesn't come with solidarity and action. Spiritual bypassing shields white women from the truth. It disconnects them and helps them avoid the big picture. It's more about checking out than checking in.*

The idea that we should spread "love and light" instead, without addressing racism and white supremacy, is really just an attempt to forgo the realities of the trauma that people are experiencing.

Focusing on love and light without acknowledging racism and its effect on the mental and emotional health of

BIPOC minimizes and disregards the trauma being experienced. Engaging in a wellness culture that emphasizes positivity to the exclusion of any other reality dismisses the fact that some of us face difficult things nearly every single day, and we can't always choose to ignore them in favor of love and light. I don't care how anyone tries to spin it. You can't love your way out of racism. You can't love your way out of systemic oppression. You can't love your way out of people's anti-fat bias. It's just not possible. Nor is it possible to have collective liberation under these conditions.

It often seems like people either just want to ignore the pain being experienced by BIPOC or put it on full display for their own benefit. White people love to hear stories about the trauma Black folks endure. I'm repeatedly asked to share my trauma and pain in an effort for people to "learn" about the necessity of anti-racism and DEI. I was recently invited by the DEI committee of a large fitness organization to speak on a panel during Black History Month. They wanted to "build awareness of the effects of systemic racism in the industry—experienced by both fitness professionals and fitness consumers." The topics to be discussed included the lack of Black representation in fitness along with stories and examples to demonstrate generational trauma and/or ongoing racism experienced by Black fitness professionals. Not only did they not have a budget to pay me, but they wanted me to share my trauma for a predominantly white audience—during Black History Month. For starters, how does that celebrate Black history?

Our existence is not one of only trauma and pain. Our history is rich with culture, ingenuity, and joy. Second, the reason that white supremacy still exists is not because folks have not seen how detrimental it is to those it affects. It is not my job, nor is it beneficial to anyone, to put my pain on display for a white audience to learn about racism.

Social media is a fickle thing. In a world of ever-changing algorithms, BIPOC creators, already at a disadvantage, see the same dynamics play out on social platforms as well. While I often share issues related to white supremacy and racism, that's not the entirety of who I am. But I have noticed that the posts that perform the best (by social media analytics) are the ones in which I'm displaying my pain and trauma. When I'm talking about the violence or hurt I've experienced at the hands of whiteness.

Kendra Austin, a writer and model, spoke of this very phenomenon in an Instagram post:

> "You're soooo authentic," I hear daily. And yet *their*—my audience members who are perhaps fairer, thinner, and more privileged—perception of my authenticity seems to only include the half of me which remains wounded and dragging behind me. Not the half of me which rejoices in the glory of having arrived in my own body and peace of mind. In the case of fat, queer, and Black storytellers, visibility often requires exploiting our deepest insecurities, even those we no longer relate to, for the sake of performing "authenticity." When will society's idea of

authenticity include embodiment of wholeness? When will that be worthy of visibility? It occurs to me, in my limited experience as a public-facing person with several marginalized identities, that the value of visibility is dictated by what exactly the audience cheers for. Many of the audiences consuming Black creation, fat creation, queer creation, are here for the show of hurt. They are here to see us perform suffering, to see us hemorrhage energy to demand respect, and to see us remain stunted in the despair of privileges that will never be. That is not my story. Suffering is not my brave tale.

Nearly three years after the events of 2020, I don't even think I recognized the impact this period had on me. To be thrust into training white folks, primarily, about racism because they were having their own personal awakening while we have been experiencing this for the entirety of our existence is a weird juxtaposition. Imagine trying to help people understand they have privilege while simultaneously harboring so much anger because multiple Black people have just been murdered again.

To further complicate the matter, the trauma I experienced was often at the hands of members of the dominant group, the same group I was attempting to educate. This trauma loop necessitates that individuals doing this work are prioritizing their self-care and finding ways to protect their mental health while also working for collective Black liberation. I wish I had all the answers on how to do a better job of prioritizing self-care, mental health, and joy while working toward liberation as a Black woman, but here are the things that have been helpful for me:

1. Therapy (with a Black woman therapist)

2. Intentional rest (without guilt)

3. Refusing to argue with white folks (about anything)

4. Acknowledging that the pain and anger I'm experiencing are valid

5. Finding refuge with other Black women to process emotions and feelings

6. Prioritizing self-care (in meaningful ways)

7. Saying "HELL NO" to people, things, and opportunities that don't align with my values or support collective liberation

8. Recognizing that it's not my job to convince white people to be less racist

My life is more than pain and suffering. My life's work is more than educating others about white supremacy. My life is joy and light and peace and love and so much more. That goes not only for me but for all BIPOC individuals, especially those with multiple intersectional identities. I will likely encounter hundreds more Annies, and people like her, in my lifetime, but my request is that you choose not to be like Annie. That you engage with anti-racism with the intention of being committed to dismantling white supremacy. That you do your best not to cause more harm to the very individuals leading you on your anti-racist journey. That you stop expecting members of historically excluded communities to share their trauma for your consumption. That you pay people equitably (and generously) for their time.

From Principle to Practice

—

1. How have you minimized or disregarded the impact of anti-Blackness in wellness culture?

2. Do you expect BIPOC, specifically Black women, to educate you about racism for free?

3. Do you enter environments and expect Black people to share their trauma with you so that you can learn about the perils of white supremacy?

4. What are some of the assumptions and stereotypes you have made about Black people and other people of color?

5. Have you expected Black educators to tone-police themselves to make your education and learning more comfortable?

6. How have you allowed toxic positivity to be a barrier to collective liberation?

7. If you're BIPOC, how are you holding space for self-care?

CHAPTER 7

Embracing Pleasure and Revolutionizing Our Relationship with Ourselves:

Celebrating How Far You've Come and Embodying the Joy of Body Liberation

I RECENTLY WENT SNOWBOARDING FOR THE FIRST TIME EVER IN my entire life, and I went with a complete group of strangers. Seriously. One day I was chilling at home doing some writing, and I got an email from someone I didn't know asking if I wanted to go on an all-expenses-paid snowboarding trip with Burton, a snowboarding gear company, in Aspen, Colorado, in ten days. I know that sounds too good to be true. A no-strings-attached trip, and they were going to pay for everything, including the snowboarding gear? I hurriedly replied yes, even though I really wanted to write, "Hell yeah," and notified my family, whom I was supposed to be visiting that same weekend, that I would have to reschedule because Aspen was calling my name.

Within two days, Burton had booked a me a flight and a hotel room and sent me to their local store in Manhattan to pick up all the gear I would need for the trip. The next Friday, I flew to Aspen to meet up with what turned out to be approximately forty other people for an amazing weekend. They ended up being a group of really badass, cool people: world-class snowboarders, NFL players, and musicians—and me, the writer. Here's what you know about the old me: I probably wouldn't have gone. I would have questioned why they were offering me this opportunity. I would have been self-conscious about not knowing anyone. I would have worried about what people were going to think about my body. I would have been worried because I didn't know how to snowboard. I would have gotten frustrated when I went shopping for gear and had a hard time finding things that fit well. I would have immediately thought I was too fat to go on the trip if I couldn't even find clothes that fit well. I wouldn't have realized that the lack of larger sizes available was the problem, not my body. Honestly, I would have just felt like I didn't belong there.

But that was the old me. The liberated me is different. I am serious about loving myself, something else that didn't happen overnight, and didn't happen without teachers to guide me along the way. Like bell hooks, who taught me so much about love and loving others and loving myself. One of my favorite books ever is *All about Love*. I've read it so many times I've lost count now, and every time I walk away not only grateful that bell hooks shared her magic with us but also inspired to fall more deeply in love with myself.

My personal ideology is that we all should fall deeply in love with ourselves—unapologetically, unabashedly, and wholeheartedly. My goal every day is to walk through life with what I call "main-character energy." Now, there are lots of interpretations of what this means, and there really isn't a right or wrong one, so I'm going to tell you what *I* mean when I say it. When I refer to "main-character energy," I'm simply saying that I'm centered on myself as the main character in my life, and I think I'm an amazing main character. I think I'm loving, caring, talented, confident, and generous, among other things. I believe I deserve to be in every room that I'm in and that opportunities come to me because I'm ready for them. I'm not going to pretend I wake up every single day and feel like I'm crushing life, because that would be a lie, but I strive to feel like that every day. Crushing life doesn't mean I'm hyperfocused on productivity or accomplishment; it means I'm happy and content and proud of the person I am. I delight in the person I am, and am working to create a life filled with joy, inner peace, abundance, aliveness, and, of course, self-love.

———

WHEN I WAS A KID, LIKE PROBABLY AROUND SEVEN OR EIGHT years old, I proudly exclaimed to my mother, "I'm just so full of myself. I just love myself so much." My mom still teases me about that to this day. I mean, yes, it's funny, but really that was the right energy. Why should we not be full of ourselves? Why should we not love ourselves so much? Somewhere along the way, many of us started to feel as if being deeply in love with ourselves and relishing in our amazingness, and being loud and proud about it, meant that we were self-centered or perhaps braggadocious or conceited. But that's so far from the truth. Radically loving ourselves is our birthright. When I'm speaking about self-love, I'm not even speaking to just how you feel about your body. I feel like the concept of self-love has been watered down and only used to describe how we feel about our bodies. I'm speaking to how you feel about your whole essence and being. Remember, we are so much more than our bodies, even though so often the conversation about self-love revolves around embracing the parts of ourselves we don't like physically. This body is just the vessel that allows us to have this human experience. It's just a shell that will eventually fade away. So I want you to fall in love with all of yourself—mind, body, and spirit.

And despite that, I'm also very realistic, and the truth is, loving ourselves is challenging. We all have that nagging voice in our heads: judging ourselves, comparing ourselves, wishing something about ourselves was different. In *All about Love*, hooks even acknowledges this, saying, "It is no easy task to be self-loving. Simple axioms that make self-love sound easy only make matters worse. It leaves many people wondering why, if it were so easy, they continue to be trapped by feelings of low self-esteem or self-hatred."

I don't know exactly when I stopped being "so full of myself." But it definitely happened. Something happened to most of us along the way that led to the demise of the self-love we perhaps felt as a child. We started getting messages that we weren't enough. That we were insufficient in some way. We started comparing ourselves with our friends and to the images we started seeing on TV, and perhaps the image we saw reflected back in the mirror didn't match what was being sold to us as beautiful. I spent well over a decade feeling unworthy.

But one day, I started getting sick of my own shit, and more importantly, I got sick of society's shit, trying to convince myself I needed to look like this or that or be like this or that, most of which was unattainable for me anyway. As a five-foot-eleven Black woman whose natural hair grows out of my head kinky and coily, I will never meet Eurocentric standards of beauty, so I decided to dismiss those standards and anyone and everyone who wanted to convince me that I needed to conform. I could spend my life trying to fit in, or I could decide to love myself for exactly who I was and embrace that main-character energy. I chose the latter. It wasn't that I flipped the switch overnight, but I started doing small things that perhaps felt out of my comfort zone.

A few years ago, I posted a picture of my sister and I in the park after finishing a workout. Both my sister and I are wearing sports bras, proudly showcasing our bodies. The caption read:

It's that time of the year where everyone is attempting to profit from our insecurities by telling us we better get our bodies "summer ready." So I figured it was the perfect time to show you a picture of me and my sister out and about in our "summer bodies." From the bottom of my heart, I want you to know that your body is "summer ready" right now. It's summer and you have a body. Tada . . . you're summer body ready. #ThisBodyIsSummerReady. One of the things I'm always striving towards is unapologetically embracing my body as it is right now in this moment. Because wishing for what used to be or what could be in the future, just keeps me dissatisfied and prevents me from experiencing joy in the present. What you don't see here are 6 pack abs or super lean bodies. What you do see is two Black girls unapologetically owning our bodies. There was a time I wouldn't dare work out with my shirt off (especially in public) because I didn't think I was lean enough. But here's the thing, there's no point at which you look "good enough" to take your shirt off. You know when you can take your shirt off? Whenever you feel like it. You know when you can wear shorts? Whenever you feel like it. You know when you can wear a bikini? Whenever you feel like it. We may not look like the women you see on the cover of fitness magazines due to the state of the fitness industry—the fatphobia, the ableism, the racism, diet culture and on and on. But we are an example of fitness because "fitness" is not a size or shape or look.

When I posted the picture and the caption, I never thought it would be so impactful for so many people. I never thought it would lead to a story about me and the post in *Shape* magazine. I just wanted to talk about the subtle changes I had been making myself, things that had previously felt uncomfortable—like working out sans shirt. I just wanted my little corner of the internet to see Black women with normal bodies, doing normal things like working out with sports bras on.

It also felt important for me to share this because one thing I had come to realize is that even if and when I decided to be happy with myself without condition or qualification, that didn't mean that everyone else was going to feel the same. It didn't mean I wasn't going to experience pushback because I chose to unapologetically love and appreciate myself. The world was still going to have opinions, and despite that, I was going to keep choosing to love myself. When you have the audacity to be comfortable with who you are and take up space, you're likely going to still be told all kinds of things that simply aren't true.

Too confident.

Too loud.

Too independent.

Too sexy.

Too self-assured.

Too ambitious.

Too curvy.

Too skinny.

Too big.

Too assertive.

Too Black.

Too much.

One of our greatest personal gifts is the ability to cultivate a deep love affair with ourselves. When we realize how magnificent we are, we will start to care less and less about what other people think about us.

Despite the reality that self-love doesn't fix the larger systemic issues or absolve us from dismantling systems of oppression, I don't think we should forget about the practice of self-love. In fact, I want all of us to lean into loving ourselves deeply, loudly, and proudly. It's rarely either/or in my opinion. It's usually both/and. The task of really loving ourselves is hard and won't save us from discrimination in the world, *and* it's also a worthy and necessary endeavor. Life is so short. Do we really want to spend it agonizing over everything that we aren't instead of accepting who we are? To go a little deeper, I don't even want you to just accept yourself. When I hear the word "accept," I hear the words "tolerate," "deal with," "acquiesce." I truly desire for us to more than accept ourselves. I want us to enthusiastically cherish and adore ourselves—to view ourselves with tenderness, endearment, and delight because we recognize how truly special and precious we are.

You are the only person you are with at all times, for twenty-four hours a day, 365 days a year. You are the person you spend all your time with from the moment you arrive on this planet until you take your final breath. That's why I think it's so important to cherish our relationships with ourselves. It's imperative that we learn to love ourselves. Would you spend the entirety of your life in a toxic relationship with a person who consistently berated you, called you names, or told you that you weren't good enough? Would you choose a partner who forced you to exercise to stay lean or restricted you from eating certain foods because they thought you needed to lose weight? Of course you wouldn't. You break up with that loser because they didn't treat you well. But unfortunately, we often do to ourselves the very things that we would never allow someone else to do to us. We say things to ourselves that we would never say to the people we love—berate ourselves, call ourselves names, pick ourselves apart; if we treated other people like that, no one would want to be around us. On top of that, we often spend the least amount of time nourishing and investing in our relationship with ourselves.

I'm sure you've heard of the popular book *The 5 Love Languages*, which explains that there are five ways people understand and receive emotional love: quality time, receiving gifts, words of affirmation, acts of service, and physical touch. The book focuses on how we can implement this into our romantic relationships to ensure that our partners feel loved in a way that resonates with them. That's cool. It really is. But for me, what I think is even cooler is if we think about how we like to be shown love and do that for ourselves. Like, yes, I absolutely want the people in your life to love on you hard, and you deserve that, because I truly believe we are all meant to be in community. But I also want you to love on yourself with the same—in fact more—intensity than you do the important people in your life.

The love-languages discussion will sometimes come up in conversations with friends, and they'll ask me, "So, what's your love language?" And I'll casually respond, "ALL OF THEM, OBVIOUSLY." Why should I only choose two? I like quality time. I like gifts. I like people saying nice and encouraging things to me. I love an act of service, and ya girl loves physical touch. I want it all, and I am not ashamed to admit it. So when it comes to applying this to myself, I do things for myself. For me, quality time looks like a relaxing evening reading a novel, or an afternoon in the park on a warm summer day. I regularly buy myself things I want, not necessities like toilet paper and shampoo (while important, completely boring), but things I desire to have for no other reason than I like nice things and I deserve them. I tell myself every day that I'm a smart, funny, talented, and accomplished bad bitch. I say that to myself because it's true, and I say it with my entire chest because I mean it. I recently hired someone to clean my house—an act of service for myself. And last, I love some physical touch, so I keep my vibrator charged and regularly engage in self-pleasure. These are the ways I show love to myself. Yours don't need to be the same, and I acknowledge that I have a certain level of privilege that allows me to do some of the things I listed, but we can all show ourselves the love we need in ways that fulfill us and fit in our budgets. Self-love doesn't need to be expensive.

Here are a few suggestions for each of the love languages:

QUALITY TIME

- Indulge in your favorite Netflix show
- Take a leisurely stroll
- Cozy up with a good book
- Listen to a podcast you enjoy

- Meditate

- Journal

- Take yourself on a solo date

RECEIVING GIFTS

- Buy yourself fresh flowers or a new plant

- Go shopping online or in person and treat yourself to something fun

- Buy yourself something yummy from your favorite bakery or treat yourself to a coffee or tea

- Buy yourself lessons for a new hobby

- Buy yourself a new book

- Pick up your favorite wine

- Treat yourself to a manicure or pedicure

WORDS OF AFFIRMATION

- Practice daily gratitude

- Look in the mirror and say, "Bitch, you doing a good job . . . Bitch, you doing a good job" (and if you don't understand this reference, put down the book for one sec, go to TikTok or YouTube, type in those words, and listen to the audio)

- Repeat affirmations that resonate with you

- Write yourself sticky notes about how amazing you are and leave them around your space

- Tell yourself often how much you love yourself and how proud of yourself you are

ACTS OF SERVICE

- Order takeout or take yourself to dinner

- Clean/organize your space

- Tackle some yard work

- Cook yourself a delicious meal

- Treat yourself to an Uber instead of public transportation or driving

- Make your bed in the morning

- Tackle an item on your to-do list that you've been putting off for a while

- Take a shower or bubble bath

PHYSICAL TOUCH

- Schedule a massage

- Give yourself a hug

- Give yourself a scalp massage

- Do a body scrub and moisturize with your favorite lotion or body oil

- Complete a skin-care routine

These are just some suggestions, but figuring out how to show yourself love is individual and will look different for each of us.

One of the best guides to how to be self-loving is to give ourselves the love we are often dreaming about receiving from others.

—bell hooks, *All about Love*

Loving yourself also looks like setting healthy boundaries, taking good care of yourself, going to therapy, making hard decisions that are ultimately the best for you, ending relationships, saying no to things and people and opportunities that no longer align with you, prioritizing your own well-being over the well-being of others, and trusting yourself. Loving yourself is waking up and choosing yourself day after day. It's showing yourself the same tenderness and kindness you extend toward the people in your life who are most important to you.

IN 2018, I FLEW TO BROOKLYN FROM WISCONSIN TO ATTEND A ONE-day retreat for women of color, led by my now best friend, Shirin. We were just getting to know each other at this point, but for some reason I felt really called to attend this event. When I mentioned to her that I was considering coming, she invited me to stay at her house if I decided to attend. Me, being woo woo AF sometimes, decided this was a sign, because Shirin really didn't know me that well yet, so if she invited me to stay at her house, this obviously meant I was supposed to go. During the retreat, Shirin led us through a "future you" meditation, which is essentially a twenty-minute deep meditation wherein you envision your future self. I had a very deep and very vivid meditation. In it, I was living in New York in this beautiful apartment, and get this, I was a writer—like writing books. And the real kicker: I was single. In 2018, when I had this meditation, I was still working at my corporate job, my side hustle was as an online coach/trainer, and I was very married. I never shared my experience with anyone except Shirin, and I didn't think too much of it because it was too jarring. I loved my ex deeply. How could it be possible that I would be living my life without him? I couldn't make sense of it. I thought about it for a couple of days after the event, and eventually started thinking that maybe I had fallen asleep and just had a crazy dream. I even rationalized that perhaps I didn't do the meditation right because it just seemed too unrealistic. But I couldn't shake the feeling that it had all seemed so real. Instead of continuing to ponder it, I tucked it away in a little box in my heart for safekeeping.

Fast-forward to 2020, and the unthinkable had already happened. I was separated. About six months later, through a series of events, I decided to move to Brooklyn. But really, I say that Brooklyn decided it was ready for me. I didn't really plan the move. One day I got a seemingly perfect opportunity to move, and two weeks later, I was going to be a Brooklynite. I remember being really nervous about what my family was going to think, especially my mom. I decided the best approach to break the news to my mom was to sit her down and have the conversation face-to-face. I asked to take her to lunch—something I rarely do—so she already knew something was up. At lunch, I let her know that I was moving to New York in ten days and David, my ex-husband, would not be accompanying me. Her face conveyed distress and shock, mixed with a tinge of disappointment. She didn't have a lot to say, just a few questions, but I knew that she was really hurt. I hated being the cause for it, but I knew in my heart I had to go to New York. I had to choose myself.

When I look at my life now, nearly five years after the retreat, I am the me from the future meditation. I also know that none of it would have happened had I not made a series of really hard decisions over the past three years: decisions that involved ending relationships, making choices that other folks didn't quite understand, and leaning into self-trust. Every decision I made was based in deep love for myself. I could never have predicted how this would all turn out, but I loved myself and trusted myself enough to know that however things turned out, I would be able to get through it.

For most things in life, there are no five-step processes, no guides to get you exactly where you want to go. I know we all want the answers. Give me the "how to" so I rid myself of the burden of choice once and for all. However, life doesn't actually work like that. At least that's what my therapist tells me every time I ask her to just tell me how to resolve my issues. ISN'T THAT WHAT I'M PAYING YOU FOR?! Make me better now, please and thank you. But my therapist is right, the journey to healing isn't linear. It doesn't come from a five-step process, and again, it doesn't happen overnight.

This is also true of the journey to self-love and liberation. The way that we arrive at a place of radical self-love will be different for every single one of us, and it will inevitably be harder for some of us. However, below are three tips that I believe can be useful for all of us:

1. Have compassion

When we give ourselves compassion, the tight knot of negative self-judgment starts to dissolve, replaced by a feeling of peaceful, connected acceptance—a sparkling diamond that emerges from the coal.

—Dr. Kristin Neff, associate professor
of educational psychology

Compassion is a powerful antidote to dissatisfaction with ourselves. When we can begin to hold ourselves with compassion, kindness, and care, we can begin to not only respect but also appreciate ourselves exactly as we are. It also works to lessen our feelings of body shame and reduces the amount to which our feelings of self-worth are contingent on physical appearance, especially when we recognize that we have all been dealt a difficult hand as it pertains to loving ourselves. We are truly doing the best we can. Compassion also happens to be the theme for my life.

Compassion:

- For my relationship with myself and my body

- For my relationships with other people

- For my relationship with self-worth

- For my relationship with productivity

- For my relationship with exercise

- For my relationship with food

I think about the times I was struggling with diet culture and body image and how infrequently I held myself with compassion, how rare it was for me to acknowledge that it was all really hard, and how often I let the bully inside beat me down even further.

Here's a gentle reminder:

You deserve compassion today regardless of how much or what you ate this weekend.

You deserve compassion today regardless of how much you have exercised lately.

You deserve compassion today no matter what the scale says.

You deserve compassion today regardless of how productive you have been lately.

You deserve compassion today even if you're still struggling to accept and love yourself.

Whatever you are experiencing, you deserve compassion, grace, and love.

2. Identify your needs and prioritize them

I have come to believe that caring for myself is not self-indulgent. Caring for myself is an act of survival.

—Audre Lorde

Sometimes we forget to prioritize our own needs or take the mental space to even figure out what our needs are. If you find yourself experiencing feelings of guilt around self-care or self-love, like perhaps that you're being too indulgent, I want to assure you that you can never be too indulgent with yourself. There's no such thing as loving yourself too much.

Capitalism teaches us that our value lies in our productivity and that downtime or time spent peacefully nourishing ourselves is a waste. But rest and ease are not a privilege; they are a right. Remind yourself of how great you feel when you intentionally prioritize activities that replenish you. Inevitably, you end up feeling more refreshed, more connected, more inspired, and more equipped to show up powerfully.

3. Stop expecting yourself to be perfect

> *Perfectionism is not the same thing as striving to be your best. Perfectionism is the belief that if we live perfect, look perfect, and act perfect, we can minimize or avoid the pain of blame, judgment, and shame. It's a shield. It's a twenty-ton shield that we lug around thinking it will protect us when, in fact, it's the thing that's really preventing us from taking flight.*
>
> —Brené Brown, *The Gifts of Imperfection*

We spend a lot of time looking outside ourselves for the answers. We scroll through social media looking at photoshopped and filtered pictures, immediately comparing people's highlight reels, their absolute best, to our worst. Comparison is the thief of joy. It robs us of our ability to ever be truly content, and it keeps us feeling like we are never enough.

And that's exactly the way the system was designed. It was created to keep us feeling less than. It was designed to keep us feeling like we are never enough. It's a distraction that prevents us from focusing on creating our magic in the world. When we are obsessing about the things we need to "fix," we lose sight of our purpose in life, and we certainly don't have the bandwidth to consider social justice or dismantling white supremacy.

The late, great Whitney Houston has a song titled "I'm Every Woman." Some of the lyrics go like this: "I'm every woman, it's all in me. / Anything you want done, baby, I do it naturally." I will tolerate no Whitney Houston blasphemy; however, I am going to respectfully disagree with her. I am not every woman, and it for damn sure isn't all in me. Plus, there are many, many things that don't come naturally to me. I cannot be all things or do all things, and more importantly, it's not healthy to set that expectation for myself.

When we can stop expecting perfection from ourselves and accept that making mistakes is part of our shared humanity, we can also stop beating ourselves up for every little misstep we make or for every potential "flaw" that we see in ourselves. We are our own worst critics, and it's challenging to love ourselves in the face of unrealistic expectations.

For those of you who are active on social media, this can feel especially hard, because no one will humble you and bring you back to earth faster than folks on the internet. I'm not even just talking about the trolls. I'm talking about your faithful followers who are watching everything you do, and although they love your content, they will not hesitate to call you in or call you out— whichever is to their choosing—when you make a mistake. The internet has very little grace, and cancel culture is real. However, when I decided that I was going to keep showing up on the internet, I also had to accept that I would likely get it wrong sometimes and people would tell me about it. Hell, I'm secretly terrified that I got something majorly wrong in this book and it's going to be my demise. But I've already decided that even if that's the case, I'm still gonna show myself grace, because ya girl isn't perfect (and I never will be).

In the introduction to this book, I shared the following words:

I love being Black. I love being tall. I love my body. I celebrate myself daily. I wrote this ode to myself some-time last year, and I mean it with every fiber of my being.

Sometimes I wonder how I got so lucky.
To be born so Black.
And so woman.
And so magical.
But then I stop questioning it.
Sometimes it just is what it is.

While I can now wholly embrace these words and feel that every day of my life, it took me a long time to unpack the impact of racism and white supremacy and its effect on my ability to love myself wholly and unapologetically. I do love being a Black woman, but my ability to do so day in and day out in a world that often treats us like second-class citizens is a result of cultivating self-love. I do it to save myself. Loving myself has allowed me to move into body liberation.

Self-love and body liberation are yours for the taking

too, and I believe that radical self-love allows us to move toward body liberation because it helps us embody just how worthy we are. I can honestly tell you that I truly live a life of joy now. But joy, like any other skill, requires cultivation and practice. Finding joy in your body and embracing your inherent worthiness is a choice—one that I have to make daily. There is no shortage of messages, people, and systems trying to convince us otherwise, and that's why I lean into joy for myself. I celebrate myself. I revel in my awesomeness. I cherish myself. I make it my business to enjoy life by leading with my joy. I prioritize the things that feel good for me. I pamper myself. I take myself out to lunch and dinner. I take myself on trips. I take myself to the movies. I smile boldly and unabashedly just because I feel good on the inside. I choose to be confident in myself and my body at every stage. I no longer worry about what other people think about my body. I remind myself daily that rejection is the universe's protection, so if someone doesn't like me for me, it's always a blessing.

Joy is my birthright. I don't say those words lightly. I mean them wholeheartedly, and I do my best every day to live those words and delight in myself. I rest often, which sometimes feels contradictory and difficult in the face of capitalism, but I keep practicing, because in my heart I know that I deserve all the best things life has to offer. I'm cultivating a soft, loving, and romantic life, filled with comfort and ease. The more I lean into liberation, the more readily I accept that I am worthy of those things. I'm worthy of joy. It's hard to put into words the feelings that I want to share with you, but most simply put, I bask in my own glory, knowing that I am pure magic. I hope that people see that joy in me. I hope it shines through. I hope they can look at me and feel inspired to cultivate the practice of joy in their own lives, because everything that I believe about myself belongs to you as well. I didn't get to this place overnight or with the flip of a switch. I also have days when I wake up and don't feel so amazing. But with time and practice and heaps of compassion, joy has slowly become my set point. So even when I wake up on the wrong side of the bed, as they say, and find myself in a funky mood or having a bad-body-image day, it's easier for me to find my way back to my truth—to my joy. I lovingly embrace the journey—the ups and the downs—and appreciate every single moment of it. The rainy days make the sunny days that much sweeter, and even in the midst of what feels like a storm, I can find moments of joy and gratitude for this amazing life I have cultivated for myself.

Going back to snowboarding in Aspen, I had a moment when I was surrounded by all these really cool people and almost started questioning why I got invited. But then I was like, "Duh . . . you got invited because you belong here just like everyone else." I then proceeded to spend the weekend being a pretty bad student of snowboarding, but laughing and enjoying myself all the while. I was in an absolutely gorgeous location, with stunning, sunny weather, embracing a new experience with total abandon. I didn't care if I was the worst one out there (which I completely was, for the record). I didn't care if I was in a bigger body than most of the other people (also true). I didn't care that being a writer isn't nearly as cool as being an X Games athlete or an NFL player. What I remember is taking in all the scenery and thinking, "Damn, this is really amazing, and I'm so lucky I get to be here. Look at all the places liberation has taken me, and I'm just getting started."

In the words of poet Upile Chisala,

> *One day our mothers may ask*
> *"Who do you love completely?"*
> *May we grow to respond*
> *"Ourselves. Ourselves. Our lovely selves."*

May we all embrace the energy of my seven-year-old self. May we always be full of ourselves. Today and every day. When we learn to truly love ourselves and adore ourselves deeply, we stop looking to sources outside us to make us feel whole and complete. Falling in love with yourself is truly the greatest love story of all time. May we always remember this, and may we always embrace the practice of delighting in ourselves and cultivating joy.

You aren't broken. You don't need to be fixed. You are enough. You are worthy and deserving of love right now. No matter what. You have always been and always will be worthy of love. It's not dependent on anything that you do. It's simply because you exist. Worthy. Amazing. Magical.

From Principle to Practice

---

1. What are two or three ways you can work to cultivate a deep love affair with yourself?

2. Write yourself a deep and romantic love letter. Gush over yourself. Appreciate yourself. Tell yourself how amazing you are. Tell yourself everything you would want to hear from a lover.

3. How do you like to be shown love, and how can you work toward doing that for yourself?

CHAPTER 8

Grief, Remorse, and the Mourning of Our Bodies

THE JOY I FEEL MOST OF THE TIME TODAY IS AMAZING, BUT IT CAN get complicated when I think about the past. I garnered a lot of positive attention when I was in a thinner body. People would actively comment on how amazing I looked all the time, and I can be honest about the fact that I really liked it. It made me feel good. It made me feel attractive and desirable. I liked the fact that people noticed that I worked out. I liked when people asked me if I was a trainer or asked what kind of workouts I did. I liked walking into a room full of men and knowing that they were going to pay attention to my body. It made me feel like I had an upper hand. Some people hate going to their ten-year high school reunions. I loved mine. I felt like I looked better than I did in high school, and I wanted people to notice.

One time I was on an elevator with my then-husband and this woman was trying to open a jar for her young daughter and couldn't get it open. She told her daughter to ask me because I looked really strong and fit. The young girl politely asked me to open the jar for her, and I obliged, easily opening the jar. I reveled in the fact that they had asked me to open the jar instead of my husband. In reality, I was a deeply insecure person who didn't feel worthy, and the external validation I received because of my body was a driving force in my life. I held on to it with every fiber of my being. Who would I be if I didn't exist in a body that people praised?

I have been on both sides. I have lived in a body that didn't get as much attention. I have lived in a body that had been told to lose weight by a doctor. I have lived in a body that often had a hard time finding clothes that fit it well. I have been in a body that walked out of stores frustrated and almost in tears because everything was too small. Then after years of participating in diet culture, I lived in a much smaller body, one that I still didn't think was small enough, even though I wore mostly smalls and mediums. But despite that, in this body, I always felt seen. I was always told I was beautiful by the world. That same doctor congratulated me for having lost weight and for regularly exercising. She never questioned how I lost the weight or if I had a healthy relationship with food. The number on the scale was the only thing that mattered. I lived in a body in which people praised me for my discipline and dedication to exercise and eating healthy.

But at the same time, there's something to be said about being seen by the world for your exterior but still feeling really sad and miserable on the inside. Even though I liked the attention, it's a lonely feeling to know that it's all super-ficial. It's all because of how you look. It's not because of who you are as a person. And how could it be? Most of this attention was from strangers or people I barely knew. Be-sides that, everything I was doing to keep my body small was literally draining the life out of me. Even when I real-ized that my obsession with thinness was slowly destroy-ing me, I still resisted what I already knew: I needed to break up with diet culture. I'm so glad I did, but looking back now, I still have to remind myself how important that breakup was, and why I'll never go back. Because it truly was a breakup, and for all the right reasons too.

I once dated this guy who was the absolute worst—like honestly, trash. I don't call people "trash," but his behavior was trash. I have no idea why I dealt with his crap for so long. It was toxic and disturbed my peace. And to be com-pletely honest, I knew I deserved better. I would decide to end things and vow to never go back, but somehow he would weasel his way back into my life like the sneaky little bastard that he was. I would fall for his promises (the same ones he'd broken time and time again) like a sucker and look at our past history through rose-colored glasses, hoping that things would be different this time. But y'all already know how this story goes. I always got my hopes up, and it was always more of the same bullshit. I would be left feeling stupid and disappointed, feeling bad about myself because obviously I was the idiot. I blamed myself and couldn't see at the time that I was being gaslit, manipulated, and undermined at every turn. When I finally ended the relationship for good, I felt a sense of relief, but I also felt sad about it even though it wasn't a good relationship. In the words of Alex Elle, author of *After the Rain: Gentle Reminders for Healing, Courage, and Self-Love*, "You can grieve the ending of something and also be grateful that it's over."

My experience with ending my relationship with diet culture felt in many ways super similar to ending my relationship with my douchebag boyfriend. With every new diet I tried, diet culture convinced me that this was the time it would be different. This time the weight loss would be sustainable. This time I would feel content and fulfilled. It would convince me that all the things I put my body through the last time weren't actually *that* bad. Sure, I often went to bed hungry and drank copious amounts of water and chewed entire packs of gum instead of eating food to satisfy my belly, but sometimes that's what was required. The reason my other attempts at dieting had resulted in me gaining the weight back was because I wasn't disciplined enough. I was the problem, not the diet. And similar to when I dumped my ex, when I decided to dump diet culture once and for all, I simultaneously felt a sense of relief but also sadness.

All breakups come with grief, even when the relationship needs to end. Just because someone or something (in this case, diet culture) is bad for you, doesn't mean you won't mourn it. You can miss something and still know that it's not right for you. However, letting go of things that aren't good for us also sets us free when we get to the other side of the grief.

There are stages of grief after a breakup, some of them being anger, sadness, and bargaining, among others, and usually, hopefully, ending with acceptance. During my breakup with diet culture and in the years that followed, I went through many of these stages.

Anger

When I initially began to learn how insidious diet culture is, and how companies intentionally prey on our insecurities because they want to make money off us, I was livid. Sure, prior to this I understood that capitalism can be ruthless, but this seemed wrong on so many levels. In many ways, I felt like the diet industry was breaking people down—ruining our self-esteem and convincing us that perfection was possible if we just bought the right products—all for their own self-interests, for profit. And essentially, that is what marketing has done to us. A part of me was also a little mad at myself for wasting so much time and energy trying to attain arbitrarily created standards of beauty, especially ones that were rooted in whiteness. Who was I kidding? It didn't matter how much I contorted and reconfigured, I was a Black woman. The world may never appreciate that, but why was I trying to find my confidence in a standard that was never created for women who looked like me?

Then my anger turned toward others. I was frustrated with the lack of diversity and inclusion I saw within the fitness industry. I was annoyed that no one seemed to understand that wellness is for everyone, even though the industry had long been catering to a predominantly white audience. I was irked that the wellness industry was upholding the same beauty standards and was just as complicit. It was oblivious to issues of racism, access, and intersectionality, and just how unwelcoming it was to historically excluded communities. But this was pre–George Floyd and the majority of folks just weren't interested in the conversation. I was angry with the women in the body positivity space sitting in front of mirrors and hunching over to try to accentuate their belly rolls and posting self-love messages without even understanding how and why what they were doing was harmful. I was just angry. Once I saw how diet culture, toxic fitness culture, and white supremacy were all intertwined, it couldn't be unseen.

Sadness

Diet culture robbed me of a lot for a lot of years. I was spending so much of my time and energy obsessing about my body, I didn't even have the bandwidth to think about what kind of life I wanted to create for myself or what kind of magic I wanted to put in the world. I didn't have any creative energy to give. I spent a good majority of my twenties like that, and sometimes I wonder what I could have done with those years if diet culture hadn't been wreaking its havoc on me. I think about all the things I didn't do because I was worried about what I looked like. I think of the ways I didn't put myself out there because I was convinced I wasn't worthy enough because of the size of my body. That makes me really sad when I think about it. It also makes me really sad when I think about how many people still feel that way. That's why I think the message of body liberation is so important. Oh, the things we could accomplish with millions of liberated folks walking around the world.

But I also felt sadness as I mourned the body that I didn't have anymore. While everyone's story and journey is different, breaking up with diet culture can sometimes mean that your body will change. When you stop obsessively counting calories and overexercising, there's a good chance you will gain weight. I most certainly gained weight and settled into what I call my "happy weight." It's the weight at which my body feels good. I feel healthy and strong and nourished. I have a good relationship with food and exercise. I don't restrict anything from my diet, and because of that, I don't think incessantly about any foods in particular, like I did when I made things "off limits." I trust myself again, and I don't even own a scale anymore. I feel great and, yes, my body is bigger than it used to be. If you're dealing with your own internalized fatphobia, that can be an unsettling thought. It's one thing to say there's nothing wrong with a person being in a larger body, and it's entirely different to decide that you personally are okay living in a larger body. It's similar to staying in a bad relationship because you don't want to be alone. Like you know the person sucks, but the fear of being by yourself keeps you there. But what you will find is that solitude and peace of mind are far better than bad company. Your fear about being in a larger body may be very real, because you are working on decolonizing your mind, which takes time. But trust me when I say that finding peace with your body is far better than spending the rest of your life being at war with yourself.

Still, there are difficult moments. The Memories feature on the iPhone is a real bitch, for example. You're just minding your business, living your best life, and here comes your iPhone showing you a memory from five years ago that you didn't ask to see today. Here you are, looking at a younger, possibly thinner version of yourself. In those moments, it's really easy to start longing for that version of yourself. Or feeling like you "let yourself go." Or feeling drawn back to dieting again—similar to wanting to go back to that bad ex. Missing what once was is normal, and it's no different for our bodies.

I wholeheartedly believe that we need to grieve the previous versions of ourselves. My Memories often tend to be pictures with my ex-husband *and* when I was thinner; it's a double whammy. Thanks, Apple! Just remind me of what my life used to be while I'm sitting in my apartment by myself deleting dating apps for the twelfth time. Those moments aren't always comfortable, and I'm often flooded with feelings of sadness. But at the same time, I can also realize that sadness doesn't mean I need to return to those versions of myself. And that leads us into bargaining and relapse . . .

Bargaining

Breaking up with diet culture is no easy feat. Even when we realize how insidious it is, we still sometimes feel the pull to continue to participate in the system, no matter how broken it is. We live in a patriarchal and oppressive society in which there is social capital assigned to meeting standards of beauty. Which is one of the reasons that there will be times when you may feel compelled to try to bargain with diet culture. You try to convince yourself that you can lose weight and be in a smaller body without participating in diet culture. You tell yourself that whatever plan you have, it's not even a diet. It's a lifestyle change, one that must end in weight loss, but still, not a diet. You're not even going to count calories. You're just going to eat well, work out every day, drink a gallon of water a day, read a book for ten minutes, take a five-minute cold shower, and practice daily gratitude. See!! Not a diet at all. Just a lifestyle change. Those also happen to be the rules for 75 Hard. I bring this up because 75 Hard is obviously a diet, but when I called it a diet on the internet, folks got so upset with me, arguing that it wasn't a diet but a lifestyle, that they were DM'ing and emailing me for days. For days. That's how committed folks can be to bargaining with diet culture.

Of course, bargaining with diet culture is not a logical thought, but you're in the stage of grief called bargaining. You are trying to make it make sense. But the truth is, you can't make sense of it because diet culture is always going to be harmful to both your physical and mental health.

There may even come a time when mourning the previous versions of your body becomes so unbearable that you actually relapse and run back to the comfort and familiarity of dieting. If you have done this, you're in good company. I've had many relapses in my day, trying diets briefly until I finally got so fed up and frustrated, I knew it was time to stop. The last time I decided to track macros, I didn't even make it twenty-four hours. You could say that it's because I'm too lazy now, or that I lack the discipline required, or that I just don't care enough anymore. But I don't think so. I think it's because I have experienced freedom now, and I simply can't be drawn back into shackles. But more importantly, when I find myself teetering on the edge, about to jump back into the abyss, I take meaningful time to stop and remember how miserable the woman in those pictures was. I remind myself of what I had to do to get that body and how hard it was to try to keep it. I remind myself how much those years were a haze because diet culture was in the driver's seat, not me. I wasn't in control and I didn't have freedom. I remind myself that I intentionally reclaimed my time, and even if I am mourning a previous version of myself, I don't need to go back to that. It wasn't good for me.

In those moments when I find myself looking back on those pictures and mourning the body I once had, I also remind myself that letting go also makes space for letting in. When I really let go of the desire for thinness, I gained so much. Here's what I gained:

- More mental space to create the work I wanted to share with the world

- More pleasure (with food, with my sexuality, with life in general)

- More freedom to enjoy every experience because I wasn't worried about what I looked like or what people thought about my body

- More time to do the things I liked instead of forcing myself to spend multiple hours at the gym each day

- More gratitude for all the ways in which my body shows up for me every day

- More appreciation for the functional benefits of strength training and movement

- More understanding of how inherently worthy I am simply because I exist

- More meaningful relationships with people who love me for exactly who I am because I'm showing up exactly as I am

- More ability to accept that not everyone will like me and that it's totally okay

- More confidence to take up space unapologetically

- More love for every inch of this five-foot-eleven Black, curvy body

Acceptance

Finally, we reach the stage of acceptance. This is where we find peace. The longer we sit in acceptance, the more we are able to find peace with our bodies and eventually freedom. The lingering effects of diet culture will likely still haunt us, but we also don't want it back anymore.

Breaking up diet culture and leaning into acceptance and eventually liberation allowed me to get back in tune with my body's needs and desires. I spent so many years allowing other people to tell me what to eat and how to move my body that it actually felt refreshing to incorporate this thing called joy into my eating and movement practice again.

How's that saying go? Nothing tastes as good as skinny feels. IT'S A LIE. First of all, skinny isn't a feeling, just like fat isn't a feeling. Second, when I was at my smallest, I was miserable. Last, food is delicious, and withholding from ourselves the joy and pleasure derived from eating in order to maintain western, racist standards of beauty is bullshit. Gone are the days of a bland chicken breast and rice with a side of broccoli. I was once prescribed a meal plan that required me to eat the same thing for sixty days straight. The worst part was that my post-workout meal included baked white fish (which I'm not particularly fond of), and I also had to eat a tablespoon of honey. Why honey you ask? That's a great question, but I have no idea, because I never even bothered to ask. I was so brainwashed and obsessed with my desire to be skinny, I didn't even question what this person told me to do.

When I was a child, I always used to dream of being an adult so I could stay up as late as I wanted and eat whatever I felt like. No one would be able to tell me what to do. My ten-year-old self would be very disappointed to know that I grew up only to spend years of my life letting other people tell me exactly what to eat and also at what times I should eat said meals. But I have now redeemed myself. As I write this, I'm breaking all the "rules." It's 11 p.m. and I'm sitting in my bed eating a very mediocre chocolate croissant. Yes, it's mediocre and the crumbs are all over my bed and will cut my legs throughout the entire night, but I'm living on my terms, and damn does it feel good.

And speaking of things that feel good, I finally started thinking about movement as something that can and should feel enjoyable. Diet culture has really disconnected us from the benefits of exercise that have nothing to do with weight loss. In fact, it wasn't until after I broke up with diet culture that I realized one could have a movement practice if they didn't intend to lose weight. Up until that point in my life, I had never intentionally moved my body just because. I'm not even sure that I realized that was an option. If I wasn't exercising to burn off calories or to beat my body into submission, then what was the point?

And there's a good reason I felt that way. Although the benefits of movement are vast—including reduced stress levels, improved mental health, better heart health, and better sleep, just to name a few—mainstream fitness tends to focus on exercise solely as a means to lose weight, frequently sharing the most effective workouts to burn fat. Why would I consider exercise for anything else? This is also one of the reasons I now refer to exercise as a movement practice. "Exercise," unfortunately, has a lot of negative connotations attached to it, thanks to diet culture, but a movement practice doesn't involve torturing ourselves with workouts we don't enjoy, and it doesn't need to involve the gym or weight training. Movement is just what it sounds like—moving your body. That could be yoga, surfing, biking, twerking to Meg Thee Stallion (i.e., dancing), swimming, or taking a leisurely stroll around the block, among other things. Moving just for the joy of it is super important, and you don't have to take my word for it. Kelly McGonigal, PhD, wrote a book entitled *The Joy of Movement*, in which she states the following:

> *Around the world, people who are more physically active are happier and more satisfied with their lives. This is true whether their preferred activity is walking, running, swimming, dancing, biking, playing sports, lifting weights, or practicing yoga. People who are regularly active have a stronger sense of purpose, and they experience more gratitude, love, and hope. They feel more connected to their communities, and are less likely to suffer from loneliness or become depressed.*

So I finally got back in touch with my body and started listening to what it wanted. And the truth is, as much as I loved powerlifting, I didn't love being in the gym for over two hours each workout. I really preferred to be in and out in less than an hour. Also, some days I don't feel like lifting weights. I just want to take a walk through my neighborhood in Bed-Stuy and catch a vibe looking at all the beautiful architecture. The old me would have scoffed at this idea and rejected this as a form of exercise because it didn't involve sweating and ending my workouts so exhausted I could barely move. But during acceptance, we realize that wow, life is really good without that toxic ex, and in this case, life is really good without diet culture.

I also need to talk about the elephant in the room. As I'm writing this, I also acknowledge that I hold a tremendous amount of privilege. For the most part, no one makes assumptions about my "health." Sure I have the occasional trolls on Instagram who leave comments like, "Let's see if your fat ass is still alive when you're forty or if you've croaked from a heart attack because you clearly don't care about your health." By the way, have you noticed that 99 percent of the time, trolls are faceless avatars with no followers? This is why I never respond. I'm not going to waste my time talking back to Mr., Ms., or Mx. Twitter fingers who doesn't even have the courage to show their face on the internet. The point is, fatphobia and weight stigma don't affect me on a day-to-day basis, and I absolutely benefit from thin privilege. On the flip side, I am a Black woman, and that in itself is political. I deal with more than my fair share of bullshit, and what I hope you can understand is that there's levels to this. We have to do a better job of understanding that it's a both/and situation—not either/or. I can be oppressed and privileged. That goes for all of us. Even though we are marginalized in certain aspects of our identity, it doesn't absolve us of our ability to also be the oppressor. Our privilege, or lack thereof, impacts both our experience of the world and the ways in which we are allowed to maneuver the world.

But privilege aside, I firmly believe that regardless of your shape or size or background, experiencing grief and remorse as we mourn our bodies or previous versions of ourselves is normal and something we don't talk about enough. We live in a patriarchal and oppressive system in which there is social capital assigned to meeting standards of beauty. So it's no wonder we may find ourselves still wanting to lose weight or change ourselves in some way to meet said standards of beauty. You may feel conflicted about wanting to continue participating in diet culture when deep down you know it's a result of white supremacy, designed to keep us distracted. But the reality is, thin privilege exists. People treat us differently based on the size of our bodies and our looks. And more than that, there are systemic benefits to living in a smaller body. Often, this results in us feeling guilt and shame for wanting access to the benefits that accompany residing in a smaller body.

So if you find yourself feeling particularly down and

having a hard time or sitting in guilt and shame for feeling bad about your body changing even when you know those feelings aren't actually helpful, I find it useful to do something to shift my energy. I often like to engage in physical movement and literally shake the bad feelings off.

My most preferred way of doing this is to dance. Everyone is different, but when I'm feeling anxious about something, I feel it in my chest, and dancing feels like I'm writhing and gyrating the bad feelings away. For the record, I'm not a good dancer, so it's not about how you look doing it. Honestly, the sillier the better. There's a dance called the "Bernie Lean." I had to google it because I didn't know the actual name for it, but I just know what it looks like. To do this dance, you lean your head and shoulders back pointed toward the sky, put your arms out behind your body, and flail them in the air. It looks ridiculous, but there is something about that dance that really helps me feel like I'm vibrating away the guilt and shame and bad energy that I feel sitting in my chest. If you're not familiar with the dance I'm referring to, please google it and take a minute to pause and Bernie Lean with me. If you are feeling foolish, relax into it more; really let go. Once you are laughing at yourself and flailing your arms uncontrollably, you're doing it right. But for real, it doesn't have to be the Bernie Lean, it can be any dance that helps you get out of your head and into your body.

I also like to go for a walk to clear my mind. I like to

remind myself to be grateful for what my body is able to do. What a body is able to do is going to be different for each of us. There's a level of ableism in statements like those, but we can be grateful for whatever our ability level is. When I first moved to Brooklyn in 2018, I found myself in an unfortunate housing situation involving a roommate (who was a pathological liar) and her dog, which was so aggressive it greeted me with a muzzle on the day I moved in. If it sounds like a bad combination, that's because it was. I'll save the details on that story for another time, but I will tell you that I lasted only five days in that apartment, and it culminated with me tripping down the stairs in an attempt to get away from the dog. My ankle instantly swelled to the size of a grapefruit, and I was left to hobble around NYC on crutches searching for a new apartment. It was a rough start to a new city. Just picture me crutching down the street with tears rolling down my face.

This is one of the first times I realized one of the most beautiful (and maybe sad) things about this city: You can cry anywhere, and no one even bats an eye. On the subway. In a coffee shop. At the grocery store. Walking down the street. No one—and I mean no one—is even going to look at you twice. All this to say, when I was injured, all I could do was lament on how much I took my healthy ankle for granted. I never woke up and said, "Thank you, ankle, for being so amazing and helping me walk with ease. I appreciate you so much. You are an integral part of my existence, and you don't get the credit you deserve." Never. And to be honest, every time I'm injured in some way, I vow to never take the simple things for granted again, and inevitably I always do. So I guess what I'm saying is, however you can move your body and clear your mind, I hope you take the time to appreciate it. Don't wait until you're hobbling down the streets of Brooklyn with tears streaming down your cheeks to realize how important your ankle is. Plus, movement (of all forms) does wonders for releasing feelings of guilt and shame from our bodies.

ON THE NONPHYSICAL SIDE OF THINGS, I'M A BIG FAN OF becoming your own biggest hype person, and when I'm struggling with grief and remorse over previous versions of myself, I like to pull out the pen and paper (because I'm old-school). My friends make fun of me because I still have a paper calendar. I like writing things down and I WILL NOT APOLOGIZE for it. But you don't have to actually use paper. You can do it electronically if you please (and I guess that's better for the environment too). Whatever method you choose, the exercise is simple. Make a list of *at least* ten things you like about yourself that have nothing to do with your body or the way you look. I say at least ten because once you get rolling, you'll realize you have so many things to say. There is no thing that is too great or too small to put on the list. Here are a few things from the list I just made about myself last week:

- I am ridiculously good at making scrambled eggs.

- I'm outrageously funny.

- I'm an awesome listener.

- I have excellent taste in music.

- I'm a great friend.

- My taste in books is superb.

- I'm an amazing brunch/lunch/dinner date.

- I'm gifted with words.

- I'm generous and kind.

- I care deeply for people.

Once you get rolling, I promise you won't be able to stop. I didn't even get to the part about me being a decent plant mom. Also, this is not the time to be modest. This is the time to be the most braggadocious version of yourself you can be.

My final suggestion is to write a compassionate and loving letter to yourself expressing that you know this is all really hard and that you are holding yourself with kindness, compassion, grace, and gratitude. All the things we need when we're going through a hard time. Don't forget to tell yourself how amazing you're doing at life (because you are). We are all doing the best we can in the midst of really challenging circumstances. When I think about this activity, I find it helpful to think of how someone who loves me dearly would address me, and then address myself in that same manner.

I hope you understand that if you're still in a place where you are struggling with the grief and remorse that often accompanies breaking up with diet culture, I wholeheartedly understand what you're going through because I've been there myself, and I'm sending you so much love and compassion. Be gentle and kind to yourself. This shit is hard. I want to encourage you to embrace the body you have now. Embrace it without conditions. Embrace it despite its imperfections. Embrace the rolls and the softness. Embrace the stretch marks. Embrace the muscles. Embrace the lumps and bumps. Embrace the scars. Embrace the acne. Embrace the curves. Embrace it even if you feel like it's failed you in some way. Embrace the sheer beauty of it all. After the grief and the mourning and remorse, may you remember that when all is said and done, you are here. Living. Breathing. Surviving. Thriving.

Lean into the beauty and magic that is you. You are a miracle, whole and complete.

From Principle to Practice

1. What experiences have you had that have shown you the realities of thin privilege, and how have these experiences impacted your desire to uphold standards of beauty?

2. Even though you recognize the harmful effects of diet culture, do you still struggle with finding yourself wanting to participate?

3. In what areas do you need to show yourself more compassion for your complicated relationship with food, exercise, and/or your body?

4. Consider writing a letter to yourself releasing any feelings of guilt and shame you may have.

CHAPTER 9

Boundaries and the Body

ALTHOUGH I CLEARLY STARTED JOURNALING ABOUT MY WEIGHT at an early age, my first big venture into dieting started during my junior year of high school, as I've mentioned before. I was probably sixteen or seventeen at the time. It was a weird period in my life. My parents were going through a divorce. My dad had just suddenly and unexpectedly relocated back to his hometown in the South. My mom was abruptly a single mother, trying to make ends meet on her own. I was a semi-rebellious teenager who was grappling with all the changes occurring, without a ton of support because, to be fair, everyone was trying to make sense of what was happening. My two older brothers were already out of the house, so it was just my mom, me, and my younger sister.

During this period, I also gained some weight. Maybe I was coping with food. Maybe not. I really don't remember too many of the details during this time period. A lot of it feels like a haze. I recently saw this meme on social media that read: "Me: I'm not really traumatized. Also me: I can't remember certain chunks of my life." Well, that's an interesting thought that perhaps I should discuss with my therapist. Needless to say, I can't remember if I noticed my body changing or if it bothered me. I don't remember if I was self-conscious about it. I've wracked my brain endlessly, and I can't recall any feelings.

But someone else noticed and made sure to bring it to my attention. I remember the moment vividly. At my high school, our cafeteria was located in the basement, and we had this small room we called "the yearbook room," where they sold chips, candy, cookies, etc. Supposedly the profits went to funding the yearbook, but we later found out that one of the school employees who helped facilitate it was actually stealing a lot of the proceeds. This went undiscovered for a long time, until he got greedy and stole our money for our senior trip. It was a whole debacle. Anyway, at the beginning of our lunch hour, we would crowd into the little room to buy our snacks. One particular day, I was standing in line with my friends when one of my classmates, a boy by the name of Khalif, looked at me and laughingly said, "I can see you've been eating good," referring to my weight gain. I laughed it off, but I was mortified. I'm not sure if Black girls can turn red, but if they can, I did that day. I decided at that moment to do something about my weight.

Although I had been counting calories and grams of fat as a preteen, in actuality I really didn't know a lot about what it would take to lose weight, except for trying to eat less and exercise more. However, my mom had a good friend who had just lost a significant amount of weight, and I had overheard them talking about the Atkins diet. So I did what one did back then—I drove to the bookstore and purchased a book about it. It seemed simple enough. Eat lots of meat and full-fat items and avoid the carbs. Y'all, when I say I committed to Atkins, I COMMITTED. While you can eat a variety of low-carb vegetables, for some reason I really liked cabbage, so I would have my mom make headfuls of sautéed cabbage, along with either baked or sautéed chicken breast. Eventually, I started making this meal for myself. I would buy low-carb or no-carb versions of everything. I ate pork rinds by the boatload. Anytime I wanted chips, I just grabbed some pork rinds. Here's the thing— pork rinds aren't terrible. They're not completely disgusting, but they also aren't very good. But the mind is very powerful, and diet culture is very convincing, so just like people pretend that zucchini noodles taste just like pasta, I pretended that pork rinds tasted just like chips. I also got really into the fact that I could eat *so* much candy, as long as it was sugar-free. I would drive myself to Walgreens and buy a big bag of pork rinds and a couple varieties of sugar-free candy. Sure, I couldn't eat a lot of foods I really enjoyed, like bread and pizza and fruit, but it was all worth it in my mind. My body was shrinking right before my eyes and I was eating "junk" food.

There's one thing that the Atkins people just don't talk about enough. Eating large quantities of sugar-free sweeteners like xylitol, sorbitol, and other sugar alcohols causes diarrhea. I'm not going to go into too much detail, but I had to learn this the hard way. It also gives you very bad flatulence, and let me just say . . . baby, my gas could clear out a room! I also had really bad-smelling breath, which I overcame by chewing sugar-free gum. Yes, these sound like terrible side effects, but I was on my way to getting skinny, so I told myself it was all worth it. I made some slight adjustments to the amount of sugar alcohol I was ingesting, but all in all, I stayed the course. And skinny I got. I don't remember exactly how long it took, but it wasn't super long, and I had shed about thirty pounds. I had also incorporated light exercise—walking. I think walking is great and has so many benefits. To this day, ya girl loves a good walk. But I got a little excessive, often walking six miles a day. Since I have relocated to Brooklyn and walk most places because I don't have a car, it's easy to get in three to five miles a day without even trying. But I was in high school living in Wisconsin, where people drive everywhere. I had read this article about a woman who walked ten miles a day and I remember thinking, "It would be so great if I could work my way up to ten miles a day." To be clear, I'm not demonizing walking. It's a phenomenal form of movement, but I can have these obsessive tendencies. Once I get started, I drill my hooks in and I can't let go. Why walk four miles when you can walk six? Why walk six when you can walk eight? Now that you've walked eight, you might as well take it up to ten. Do you see what I mean? Also, I wasn't walking for health. I was walking because it was helping me dwindle my body. And to be honest, when you're eating fewer than fifty net carbs a day, do you really need to walk miles and miles on top of that? That's not even enough carbs for normal brain function, much less thousands and thousands of steps.

It didn't take long for my peers to notice my new, thinner body. Everyone complimented me, told me how great I looked, begged me to share my weight-loss secrets with them. And I felt redeemed. No one could comment on my weight anymore. There was nothing to be said. I was thin. I don't know a single person who has lost weight who hasn't immediately been praised for it. And I would be lying if I didn't say I enjoyed it at the time. I liked people noticing my "new and improved" body. A lot of us probably like it initially because we have all been so ingrained with fatphobia that we accept these compliments as acknowledgment that we are in a "better" body, and if our fat loss was intentional, it's kudos for accomplishing our goal. It feels good momentarily.

However, the reality is, complimenting people on weight loss is harmful. It reinforces the narrative that smaller bodies are inherently more beautiful, more healthy, and more worthy of attention and praise. For people on the receiving end who may already be struggling with body image, it drives home the point that people prefer them in a thinner body.

We live in a culture that praises weight loss. What's the message we are sending when we say, "Wow, you look so great," in response to weight loss? Did the person not look good before? Do they look better now simply because they are in a smaller body? I have never once been showered with compliments due to weight gain. People have definitely commented on the fact that my body got bigger, but it was never complimentary. They never said, "Oh I can tell you gained some weight. Congrats! You look amazing." Nope, that's never happened.

Even hearing that now, after I've moved toward body liberation, it might sound strange because it's the polar opposite of what we're used to. The thing about fatphobia is that it's so similar to white supremacy in that unlearning it is a lifelong journey. I see anti-Blackness rear its ugly head in my life all the time and am constantly working to decolonize my belief systems and unlearn narratives that don't belong to me. Fatphobia is the same. Maybe you even heard that little voice in your head say, "But why would I congratulate someone on gaining weight?" The response to that question is, why would we congratulate people on fat loss? And the answer is simple: fatphobia. Regardless of our intent, we perpetuate diet culture and fatphobia when we compliment someone on their smaller body. It's our own biases that are showing. Our preferences for thinness, which are ingrained in white supremacy and racism, come through as compliments for the achievement of a thinner body.

Our society praises weight loss as if it's the best thing a person could possibly do. We comment on people's bodies without having any idea what is going on with them. We assume that weight loss is a *positive*. Unbeknownst to us, weight loss could be occurring because of a chronic or terminal illness, serious depression, a breakup, an eating disorder, grief, stress or anxiety, or chronic unhealthy dieting. I've talked about this numerous times on my Instagram account and gotten hundreds of DMs from people sharing their stories with me. Stories of going through some of the most difficult and traumatic periods of their lives and being congratulated on weight loss when they were, in fact, suffering terribly. Being praised for weight loss is a constant reinforcement that being thin is the best thing we can be in the world, and people like the smaller version of us better, regardless of what it went through to get smaller. Is there any wonder that so many of us spend far too much energy obsessed with shrinking our bodies?

Here's my opinion. We should never—and I mean *never*—make unsolicited comments about someone else's body. EVER. Period. It doesn't matter if we consider the comment to be good or bad. All unsolicited comments about someone's body are bad because no one asked for them. I also believe that we should never congratulate weight loss. We've all been guilty of it before. I certainly have. This is not about shaming or judging, but rather about recognizing that we have to do better as a society and a culture. In terms of both personal and collective body liberation, we can't achieve that until we learn to keep our mouths shut as it pertains to other people's bodies while simultaneously doing the work to unlearn our biases.

Refraining from commenting on other people's bodies also prevents you from making a donkey out of yourself, so it's also very sound practical advice. I have two stories about this. When I was much younger, probably in my very early twenties, I ran into a childhood friend of mine named Jennifer. We had grown up together in church and spent lots of time together over the years, but as happens in life, we grew apart and went separate ways. When I ran into Jennifer, over a decade had passed since I had last seen her. Social media had kept me in the loop enough to know she had gotten married. When I saw her, I enthusiastically said hi and gave her a hug. And then I opened my mouth and said one of the dumbest things I've ever said. "OMG, you're pregnant! Congratulations." The smile dropped from my friend's face as she quietly told me that she wasn't pregnant. I was apologetic, but what can you really say to make a moment like that less awkward? Nothing. There is nothing you can say to make it less awkward. I had put my foot in my mouth and there wasn't really a way to backpedal. She changed the subject, and we chatted a few more minutes before we wrapped up the conversation. I still cringe thinking about that incident. What I wouldn't do to go back in time and get a do-over. However, it did teach me a valuable lesson about making unsolicited comments on people's bodies. These days you could be ten months pregnant, about to pop at any moment, and I am not mentioning the baby in your stomach unless you yourself have let me know that you are pregnant. So if we ever run into each other and you're pregnant and you would like to talk about it, you will have to explicitly bring it up. I'm not being rude. It's just that I learned my lesson the hard way and that mistake is never going to happen again.

Karma is bitch though. A couple of years after this—I don't know the exact timeline—I was on the receiving end of the same situation. I was working as a bank teller while I was finishing college. It was during one of my many weight-regain cycles. An older Black woman came to my window to do her banking transaction and smiled at me with the sweetest face and proceeded to say, "You look so beautiful pregnant. When are you due?" I sheepishly replied, "I'm not pregnant." Embarrassed, she said, "It's probably your sweater that makes you look like that." I'm not sure if that was supposed to make me feel better or not, but it didn't. I was mortified and again decided it was time for another diet. I had clearly "let myself go" if I had gained so much weight that people were mistaking me for a pregnant person. In hindsight, I'm not even sure which one felt worse. Being the asshole who put their foot in their mouth or being on the receiving end of the asshole who put their foot in their mouth. They both suck. Take it from me and save yourself. Don't make unsolicited comments on someone else's body.

And you know what? Take it a step further and tell people you don't want to receive those comments either. I've seen great examples out there. In an Instagram post on October 13, 2021, actor Jonah Hill wrote the following words:

> I know you mean well but I kindly ask that you not comment on my body. Good or bad. I want to politely let you know it's not helpful and doesn't feel good. Much respect.

This, my friends, is called setting boundaries. Something that often feels difficult to do but is 100 percent necessary in life, especially when it's about something as personal as our bodies. Also, I agree with Jonah. Having people comment on our bodies doesn't feel good, nor is it helpful. How many of us have been impacted by the words other people spoke about our bodies? I'm not saying that a sixteen-year-old boy named Khalif is responsible for the years of dieting that ensued after his comment. I'm also not saying that the woman who asked me if I was pregnant is responsible for my next yo-yo diet, because I clearly had issues with my body prior to this. But what I am saying is the way people talk about our bodies can have an effect on our body image, regardless of their intention.

Because of this, it's important to set boundaries for ourselves in order to protect our own well-being in a world that may not be on the same page as us. It took me a long time to break up with diet culture, but within mainstream fitness and wellness, as well as in many of our social circles, diet culture is still rampant. Just because we individually have decided to break up with diet culture doesn't mean that everyone around us is automatically going to be on board, and thus, boundaries are needed. But what are they exactly? In the most simple form, boundaries can be defined as our list of what we consider okay or not okay as it pertains to how people engage with us and how we engage with others. In other words, it's the rules we set for our relationships. I will not pretend to be the boundary expert, because even as a thirty-six-year-old woman, I still occasionally struggle with boundary setting because it almost always involves uncomfortable conversations. But as we already covered earlier in this book, we can do hard things. So even though it's hard for me, I push through the discomfort and always feel better for having done so.

I don't pretend to have all the answers, but if you also struggle with boundary setting, especially as it pertains to your body and diet culture, here are some tips that you may find helpful.

Establish boundaries with social media

I genuinely love social media. I met my best friend and lots of other amazing people through Instagram, and I think social media allows us to connect with people all over the world who we might otherwise have never met. I've also gotten the opportunity to share my work and words in a larger capacity. It allows everyone a semi-equal playing field to share their work (if we ignore the fact that the algorithms are racist and negatively impact BIPOC and queer creators). However, for all the positives, there are also some drawbacks. One of them being the same that I just named as a positive—everyone can share their opinions.

That being said, it's the perfect environment for diet culture to flourish. It's the perfect place for us to find ourselves falling into the comparison trap. It's the perfect place for us to get inundated with before and after pictures. Diet culture thrives on the idea that certain bodies are "better" than others already. Add in Photoshop and filters to the mix, and social media has the capacity to affect anyone's self-image and sell you on the next best diet or exercise program to help you achieve "the body of your dreams." As a collective, we spend a lot of time on social media. I know I spend more time there than I care to admit. So if I'm going to be there, I think I should try to make it as healthy an environment for myself as possible. For me, that means intentionally curating my feed, which means that I'm a big fan of both the unfollow button and that mute button. If I feel triggered by content, if it makes me feel less than, if it makes me question my worth, if it makes me feel drawn back into diet culture, it's not content I want to see on my timeline.

That doesn't necessarily mean there's anything wrong with the content. It could just mean that it doesn't make me feel good based on my current circumstances, and therefore I set a boundary about seeing that content on my newsfeed. If looking at someone else's "perfect" body triggers my own body image insecurities, perhaps it's not content I need to see. That says nothing about the person or content, and everything about my choice to prioritize my own mental health. And of course, there's a vast amount of content being produced and shared that is straight up fatphobic. I don't need to see that either.

Last, there is zero reason to feel bad about unfollowing or muting folks on social media. It's your little corner of the internet. You get to choose who you want in it. If it doesn't support your well-being or bring you joy, let it go. Hell, you should unfollow me if my content no longer aligns with you or doesn't make you feel good. I won't take it personally. In fact, I'll congratulate you for choosing yourself.

Establish boundaries with friends, family, and lovers

When it comes to my friends, I'm very intentional about my circle. I want to cultivate relationships that are characterized by love, joy, respect, and reciprocity. I believe that my energy is a gift and that allowing people to access my energy is also a gift. So I'm careful about who I spend my time with. If we're friends, I want you to walk away from our interactions feeling energized, loved, and appreciated, and I want to walk away feeling the same way. One of my boundaries for friendship is that we don't engage in diet culture when we're together. That doesn't mean we don't talk about our body image struggles, because we definitely do. It means that when we're at a restaurant eating dinner, we don't talk about calories. We don't demonize food. We don't talk or make judgments about other people's bodies. We don't engage in fatphobia. We hold each other accountable. We call each other in. In order to be in my circle, you have to actively be dismantling white supremacy, racism (and other "isms"), and fatphobia from your life. We don't get to choose our biological family, but we do get to choose our friends. I have worked really hard and continue to work daily on falling deeply in love with myself and being at peace with this shell I reside in. I'm not going to allow folks in my circle who can't support that. If those boundaries can't be respected, it doesn't mean I won't love you, but I will choose to love you from a distance. Life is too short to spend it with people who don't support us in living our most actualized, diet-free lives.

Our family members can be an entirely different story altogether. Often, family members feel entitled to speak as they please about anything and everything. In BIPOC homes in particular, our family is going to let us know what they think, unabashedly. Aunties, grandmas, cousins, whoever, will often freely greet you at the door with commentary about your body. These situations can be more delicate and difficult to navigate. Because of certain family dynamics and the ways we honor our elders in our respective families, there's no cut-and-dry way to handle this (or at least not that I feel comfortable giving my thoughts on). This is one of the reasons I have a Black therapist. My therapist understands the dynamics of a Black family and will not automatically suggest that I cut off Auntie Barbara for calling me fat. I'm not saying it's not okay to cut family members off, but I'm saying that sometimes it's far more nuanced, and for BIPOC, our respective cultures potentially play a role in how we navigate this terrain.

When I previously did one-on-one coaching, one of my clients knew that spending time with her mother was going to trigger her body image issues. Her mom struggled tremendously with her own body image and held a lot of biases about bodies, so my client knew that whenever she saw her mom, her mother was going to bring up both of their weights, talk about diet possibilities, and demonize their food choices. After having countless conversations with her mom expressing that we wanted to set boundaries about the amount of diet talk that occurred when they were together and seeing no changed behavior on behalf of her mom, my client decided to accept that her mom wasn't likely to change anytime soon. She had no interest in cutting her mom off, but also realized that after every visit with her mom, she left upset, frustrated, and feeling bad about her body. My client decided to do two things to protect her own well-being. For one, she still visited her mom, but she chose to go less frequently. Second, she spent more intentional time before each visit working on her own mindset and showing herself some extra love. Post-visit, she made sure to give herself a generous amount of compassion. Over time, she was also able to internalize less of the body talk that occurred when she visited.

We also may consider that perhaps we only see certain family members around the holidays or for special occasions, so we set boundaries about how much time we spend with the people who feel a little too comfortable commenting on our bodies or engaging in diet talk. Maybe our boundary is that we are going to spend two hours at the family function and then head on our merry way. Ultimately, we individually have to decide what is best for us.

Last, when it comes to lovers and romantic partners, it's simple. I am a gift. I am the prize. I will accept nothing less than absolute worship of my essence, being, and body. If my body is not to the liking of a romantic partner, they can see themselves out. The world already has enough to say about our bodies, I don't need to deal with it in the bedroom too. I'm only interested in romantic partners to add to my ability to love and cherish myself. For the record, I am not advising you on what to do with your partner, and I am by no means suggesting you break up with your partner via text right now. I'm only telling you the boundaries I have for people I'm romantically involved with. You can do with that information what you will.

As much as we love our friends and loved ones, there's a good chance our boundaries will be challenged at some point. Nedra Glover Tawwab, therapist and author of *Set Boundaries, Find Peace*, offers some amazing ways to respond when we find ourselves in situations in which people we care about are challenging our boundaries:

"I'm changing, and this is what I need now."

"This is not negotiable."

"We think differently about this, and I don't want to argue about what feels healthy for me."

"It's okay if you don't like what I'm saying, and I need you to respect it."

"I mentioned this as a solution because I want to maintain the relationship."

Here are a few of my suggestions:

"My body and my health are not up for discussion. Thank you for respecting my feelings."

"I want to continue spending time with you, but I don't want dieting and weight loss to be part of our conversations."

"I understand that you are just expressing your concern, but I don't want to discuss my choices about food."

"I know you probably don't have bad intentions, but it makes me uncomfortable when you comment on my body, so I would appreciate it if you would refrain from doing that."

Establish boundaries with your doctor

My well-being is my priority. I know that the scale can be a trigger for me. Even though I know that the scale is just a number, it can still set me off sometimes. When I go to the doctor, I either ask not to be weighed (which is my right and rarely medically necessary) or I inform them that I'm turning around because I don't want to see the number. I also make it a point to inform the nurse and doctor that

I don't want that number discussed during my appointment, even if they think it's a positive, as in the number went down since my last visit and they want to congratulate me. That's a firm no for me. No diet culture, please.

Doctors can be intimidating in general. Even more so if you are in a larger body. Do whatever you can to find a provider you feel most comfortable with and believe is invested in actually hearing you. As a Black woman, I always have to advocate for myself when it comes to healthcare, and a boundary for me is that I want my primary care provider to be a Black woman, or at least a person of color if a Black woman is not available for some reason.

DESPITE ALL OUR BEST EFFORTS, WE WILL STILL SOMETIMES FIND ourselves in social situations where diet culture and fatphobia rears its ugly head—at work, at parties, etc. In those situations, I usually do one of the following:

1. Change the subject

If we are eating appetizers at a party and someone says, "OMG, this is going to go straight to my waistline," and everyone quickly chimes in expressing more of the same, I might just interject a completely different topic altogether. If I was in this situation today, I would say something like, "Did y'all watch *The Tinder Swindler* on Netflix yet? Wasn't that story wild?!" If you've seen it, then you know this is the perfect distraction to a conversation about diet culture. Use whatever current show is the talk of the time and move on to entirely frivolous conversation.

2. Walk away

Sometimes I just don't have the bandwidth or desire to confront someone, so I simply excuse myself from the conversation and find someone else to engage with, or I go to the restroom. That's honestly as easy as it gets.

3. Ignore it altogether

Sometimes I choose to just let the conversation happen and not engage personally. Energy is a limited resource, and I pick and choose when I want to shoulder the burden. It's the same as conversations about racism. It's not my job as a Black woman to educate every person I meet about why what they just said was racist. It's too large a burden to bear. For folks with multiple intersecting identities, sometimes you may not have the energy or the desire to be the educator, and choosing to not engage may be the best choice for your well-being and mental health. For individuals with more privilege (white, thinner-bodied folks), I encourage you to take these opportunities and be a co-conspirator.

4. Take the time to educate or reframe the conversation

I often take these opportunities to push back and talk about how I have done a lot of work dismantling my own fatphobia and biases and explain how they both color our perceptions about bodies. I will also share book recommendations for folks to do the work to learn more. Along the same lines as above, I am not a resource. I am a Black woman who has done a lot of my own unlearning and education, and after some explanation, I compassionately suggest and encourage folks to do the same for themselves. I will also repeat the same for my white friends who want to act as co-conspirators. As you learn, share the knowledge you have acquired and actively be a disruptor, particularly with your own people. (This isn't an invitation to use your newfound knowledge to police members of historically excluded communities; use it to educate members of your own community—i.e., talk to your white friends.)

I WON'T PRETEND THAT ALL THE THINGS WE JUST DISCUSSED ARE easy, because that would be a lie. However, we are allowed to set boundaries with those closest to us in order to maintain agency and autonomy over our bodies. Our bodies, our business.

ON VALENTINE'S DAY OF THIS YEAR, MY BEST FRIEND SURPRISED me with the most amazing love letter in which she gushed about how amazing I am. If that's not enough, she read it to me over Zoom and recorded it for her podcast. Here is an excerpt from it:

> *You have shown me what courage is. From completely uprooting your life and moving to New York to be a writer to the things you do in your day-to-day life, you are courage embodied. Courage means to speak from and act from the heart. And that is what you do each and every day. From the words you write, to the words you speak, to the way you live your life. It is always from your heart. You have one of the biggest hearts I have ever encountered. Your capacity to love is so great. And I am so grateful that I get to bask in the glow of your heart. It's an amazing place to be. I feel so privileged to be here. I have seen your journey up close and I know it hasn't been an easy ride all the time. But you have always risen above and beyond. We joke that you are able to manifest whatever it is you desire— and you know this is true. It's because of your un- wavering belief in yourself and your life. Your desire for better, for more, for everything you desire inspires me so much.*

This is one of the most meaningful letters I have ever gotten from a friend and every compliment in it meant so much to me. Courageous. Loving. Inspiring. Those are all amazing attributes to have someone speak about you. The letter brought me to tears, and the most noticeable thing about this love letter is that it included absolutely nothing about the size of my body or how I look. It's so, so much better than being complimented based on someone's biased standards of how my body should look, which is lazy, boring, and unoriginal. It takes zero effort, nor does it say anything about the person I am.

There are so many other and, in my opinion, more interesting ways to compliment people without talking about their looks or their bodies. Here is a list of ways to hype up your friends without participating in diet culture:

"You always make me laugh, and I love spending time with you."

"You are rocking that outfit. It looks great on you!"

"You have the best smile."

"You're such a great listener."

"You're so thoughtful."

"I feel so blessed to have you in my life."

"You're so talented."

"You inspire me."

"You have such great style."

"You make my life so much better."

"You're so strong."

"I love the way you bring joy to every room you're in."

*"You're so reliable, and that means a
lot to me."*

"You're such a special person."

"You're so smart."

"You're such a good _____."

"I love your energy."

"You give the best gifts."

"That color looks great on you."

"You have a beautiful mind, and I love our conversations."

"I love your work."

The options go on and on, and I don't know about you, but these feel so much more meaningful than someone complimenting me on my body. To be fair, I'm not saying that we should never tell our loved ones they are beautiful. I love a compliment like that from an intimate relationship— platonic or romantic. However, I do think we should steer clear of giving unsolicited comments on people's bodies, especially as it pertains to the size of someone's body.

In a world that focuses too much on the physical body, we can empower one another by choosing to center who we are, not what we look like, in our day-to-day interactions. Don't be the friend who comments on someone's weight or someone who makes assumptions like I did all those years ago. Instead, be like my best friend and compliment someone for who they really are, empowering others to feel good about their authentic selves. Sometimes we think these small actions aren't that important, but they are, and each drop in the bucket is helping us all move toward body liberation.

From Principle to Practice

---

1. How have you judged people, women in particular, based on their looks?

2. Do you compliment people on weight loss without recognizing how this is participating in diet culture and upholding patriarchal standards of beauty, even if you have the best intent?

3. What biases do you hold about bodies? About Black bodies? About trans bodies? About women's bodies?

4. Make a list of ten to twenty ways to encourage and uplift people without discussing their bodies.

5. For the next week, take note of every time you make assumptions, judgments, or comments about other people's bodies.

CHAPTER 10

Love, Dating, and Body Liberation:
Our Bodies Are Not the Measure of Our Worth

I'LL LET YOU IN ON A LITTLE SECRET. I MEAN, TECHNICALLY IT'S not a secret, but it's not something that I've talked about publicly, unless you listen to the podcast I have with my best friend, *Two Girls Talking Shit*. And due to our general lack of dedication when it comes to the podcast, I'm guessing you haven't, but I promise that it's really great and you should go listen now (well, after you finish reading this). I got married at the tender age of twenty-two. In hindsight, I was far too young. But nonetheless, I was married to a wonderful man, and we spent eleven years married. We didn't end in some bitter, tragic debacle. In fact, it probably was one of the most amicable divorces of all time, and we remain good friends to this day. He's an amazing human. But all that to say, since we started dating at the age of nineteen, I had very little dating experience when our marriage ended. Just the thought of being in the dating world as a grown-ass woman was enough to elicit the same feeling I get when I'm peering over the edge of a railing of anything even remotely high. Sure, it's not really dangerous per se, but just the thought that I *could* accidentally slip and fall to a tragic death is enough for me.

One of the things I never anticipated was how much entering the dating scene at the age of thirty-four would trigger my body image issues. As I have already stated, body liberation doesn't mean that you will never again have a negative body image. In fact, due to the preponderance of messaging we receive about our bodies, I think there will always be instances where our body insecurities rise to the surface. I realize that's not a comfortable thought, but it's a realistic one. And if anything will trigger body insecurities, it's the thought of getting naked in front of cisgender, heterosexual men after being with the same person for approximately fourteen years. Yikes.

It was during the beginning of 2020, right after the pandemic started and we were in full-on lockdown, that I decided to enter the world of online dating. I know—it was an odd time to start online dating, when the world had literally just shut down. But I guess it's because I no longer had the luxury of meeting people in person (mixed with sheer boredom) that led me to this decision. Prior to this, I honestly hadn't been too concerned with dating in general. I had moved to New York from Wisconsin just six months prior to this, so honestly, acclimating to my new single life in a completely different environment was more than enough for me to focus on. I had bigger fish to fry than men. But now I found myself locked in my house, bored, lonely, and antsy. And so online dating it was.

One of the first men I connected with ended up being a man that I went on to date for several months. You know those situations when you look at a person, see all their potential, and decide to ignore the mountain of red flags that are trying to get your attention? They were basically yelling at me at the top of their lungs and begging me to stop moving forward. I would love to tell you that I'm too smart to get myself in a situation like this, but alas, I'm not, and I ignored all those red flags. So many. I'm going to blame it on my general lack of dating experience and the god-awful pandemic that was plaguing the world. If you've ever found yourself in a similar situation, I hope you find comfort in knowing that it happens to the best of us.

Needless to say, after about five or six months, I came to my senses, ended things, and ceased all communication. A couple months later, this person reached out to apologize for his poor behavior. When I didn't reciprocate in the manner he wanted, this person, who, by the way, claimed to be a "changed" individual, grew increasingly more agitated, threatened to sue me if I used any pictures he took of me (he was a professional photographer, and honestly, that's pretty much the only thing I missed: the free pictures; shoulder shrug—what can I say, it's the truth), and finally sent me one last text before I blocked him. It read:

Go fuck yourself you obese bitch

Well, if that didn't confirm one of my worst fears about dating—that someone would think my body wasn't good enough. And that didn't come from nowhere. The reality is that even if and when we are comfortable in our own skin, we still exist in a society that often *does* judge us based on our bodies.

However, it turns out it didn't faze me as much as I thought it might have. Yes, it angered me because of the utter disrespect and the audacity of this man. Like the actual audacity. I'm not one to toot my own horn, but *toot toot*. I'm a bad bitch, if I do say so myself (and not because of how I look, even though I am cute as hell, but because of who I am). How dare you, sir? For real, how dare you?! But more than anything, it reminded me of how fatphobic people are. The fact that the *worst* thing he thought he could call me is a fat bitch is indicative of the culture we live in. This person was intimately familiar with the work I do around body liberation as well as with my past body image issues, which made it even worse that angry, anti-fat bias was his venom of choice.

Because I always attempt to be cognizant of proximity to privilege, it's not lost on me that I'm a heterosexual, cisgender, straight-size woman. If I have to deal with that type of disrespect, what does that mean for individuals with additional multiple intersecting identities or for people in bodies larger than mine?

And as evidenced by the experience I just told you about, it's not uncommon for people to defer to making disparaging comments about our bodies and our looks when they want to insult us. We have all been indoctrinated to believe that being smaller is indicative of our worthiness. As I've already told you, even at my absolute leanest, I was still unhappy. I looked in the mirror and saw everything that was wrong with me. It didn't matter how much external validation I received. It didn't change the way I felt, because my personal idea of worthiness was still connected to what I looked like, and at the time, I felt valuable, beautiful, and worthy of adoration only if I was in a thin body. There was always five more pounds to lose. I would lose those five pounds and then it would be five more pounds. And if it wasn't more pounds, it was something else. A bigger butt. A smaller waist. More defined arms. Less defined arms. A flatter stomach. Smaller hips. Slightly bigger hips. The harsh reality is that you can't diet your way out of hating yourself or into loving yourself. Once you take all the measures to lose the weight—the restrictive diets, the overexercising, the sacrificing of your sanity, whatever you need to do to get smaller—you will still be the same person you were running from, just in a smaller version. That's one of the biggest lies of diet culture. That happiness is on the other side of fat loss. It leads you to believe that the empty, dull ache you're experiencing deep in your soul is going to be transformed. But being in a smaller body does not dull that ache. We have to actually address what is causing that ache, and it normally goes beyond just the scale and our negative relationship with our bodies.

I never attempt to speak for everyone, nor am I pretentious enough to think that my experience must be similar to others', but I can tell you from personal experience that the times I feel most called to fat loss or dieting is when other things in my world feel out of control. When I'm feeling emotionally out of sorts or going through a particularly difficult time, especially when I'm in a situation I can't control, diet culture rears its deceptive head, pretending that it can be the solution to all my problems.

IN 2019, IT FELT LIKE MY WORLD HAD FALLEN APART. I MENTIONED earlier that my long-term relationship ended. But what I didn't mention is that two weeks after that, my dad tragically and unexpectedly passed away. It was one of the most devastating blows in my life up to that point. Nothing really prepares you for the grief of ending a fourteen-year relationship, followed by the sudden and unexpected death of your father. That's the kind of grief that knocks you out. The kind of grief that leaves you spiraling and grasping for something to hang on to. I was spiraling in a cycle of guilt, shame, and remorse. Nothing made sense to me at that point, and I was left questioning, asking what the point of anything was. I won't lie to you and pretend that I'm great with handling feelings and emotions, because I'm not. I mostly want all the feelings to just go away. I want to skip the part where you sit with them and process them. The middle is messy and mostly uncomfortable. I want to be at the end, on a path flourishing with roses and glimmering with rays of sunshine.

Needless to say, the thought that kept coming to my mind was that I should lose some weight. Maybe that sounds ridiculous to you, considering all I've told you about my journey. It kind of does to me, but the more and more I think about it, it doesn't sound that ridiculous. My life felt in shambles at that point, and the dominant thought haunting my mind was about shrinking my body, something I could control, and something I'd controlled before. I really think that weight loss is a crutch sometimes. Focusing on weight loss, "fixing" our bodies, sometimes feels easier than addressing the deep emotional wounds or traumas we have. Sure, I could do the deep work to heal, which would likely involve therapy, ugly cries, sitting with loneliness, screaming into pillows, and exploring my feelings. Or I could focus on the things that felt far more in my control and, if I'm being honest, less painful: Get on an exercise plan—in the name of "health," of course—and eat "better" and look the best I can (according to cultural standards of beauty and diet culture). Trying to control our bodies is not the answer to the emotional pain we may be experiencing in other areas of our lives, but it often feels like it could be.

There was also a moment after I received the "Go fuck yourself you obese bitch" text that I did question my body. I wish I could tell you that the thought never crossed my mind, but it did. Not even so much because I truly thought something was wrong with my body, but more because I thought that being in a smaller body would perhaps protect me from ever experiencing hurtful comments like that again. I don't think I'm alone in this thought. Do you know anyone who experienced a painful breakup and decided to lose weight and get in the best shape of their life? I bet you do.

Isn't that what the concept of a "revenge body" is all about? The term "revenge body" has been used to describe getting a "better" (insert "smaller" or "leaner") body to demonstrate to your ex, especially if they cheated or ended the relationship with you, that you're doing better without them. We often hear this term thrust upon celebrities after breakups, but it's commonplace for people to discuss themselves in this manner now. On Instagram, there are more than 150,000 posts using the hashtag #RevengeBody. It's the idea that you are going to level up your body and appearance and show your ex, or perhaps anyone who's mistreated or hurt you, what they're missing out on or how big of a mistake they made by leaving you or treating you badly.

Western culture has put a huge emphasis on bodies, especially the bodies of women, and the idea that the body is a direct reflection of our worth and worthiness, especially as it pertains to our sexuality and desirability. The concept of a revenge body solidifies this idea. In 2017, Khloé Kardashian, who has publicly and openly struggled with body image, even launched a reality-TV show entitled *Revenge Body*, which pairs individuals up with celebrity trainers, nutritionists, and stylists to help people build their revenge bodies. In one of the trailers for the show, two people are showcased: one whose boyfriend said he was no longer attracted to him because he had gained weight, and another woman who was tired of being the DUFF (designated ugly fat friend—her words, not mine) in her friend group.

Both participants worked out seven days a week, twice a day, for the duration of thirty days. At the end of the thirty days, they revealed their new revenge bodies to their loved ones. The self-proclaimed DUFF said of the experience, "This has changed who I was, who I am, who I will ever be." My heart hurt a little bit when I heard her say this, because I've believed those words before. I've felt that way before. There was a point in time when I truly believed that I could love myself and my life more if I was in a smaller body.

I don't blame either of these individuals for participating in a show designed to help them create their revenge bodies. They aren't to blame. I don't even blame Khloé Kardashian. She's a victim just like all of us. Plus, consider all the public humiliation Tristan Thompson has put her through. It's not the time to pile on. But seriously, diet culture is always to blame, not the individual. However, if I could share a message with these two people, it wouldn't be about how terrible diet culture is (even though it is really terrible) or even that I'm so sorry they put their bodies through so much torture for thirty days (even though I am really sorry, because I've been there and done that and know the havoc it wreaks).

I would simply share my own personal experience with fat loss and body change. That getting smaller didn't help me actually feel better about myself or more worthy of love. Because the truth is, the measure of our worth does not come from our external appearances. It's not the size of our waistlines or thighs or our beauty that defines us. The reality is that if we base our self-worth on something as ever-changing as our bodies, we will forever be on the emotional roller coaster of body obsession and shame.

When I was confronted with the harsh reality that changing my body didn't in fact make me feel better about myself, I had to face the truth. I didn't really know where I was deriving my self-worth. And the more I thought about it, the more I realized it was coming from really fickle and ever-changing aspects of my life—the size of my body, my career, how much money I had in the bank, and even and especially my relationship status. Things that are rarely static and often out of our control, even if we like to believe the contrary.

Have you ever really stopped to think about where you're deriving your worthiness from? Like truly stopped to inter- rogate it? I know I didn't for a really long time, but as I started having realizations about my self-worth, I started asking myself some tough questions and compassionately sitting with the answers. What was truly making me feel worthy?

I want you to take a few minutes to ask yourself the following questions:

What's making me feel worthy?

Is it the number on the scale?

Is it the size of my jeans or other clothing?

Is it the amount of weight I can lift in the gym?

Is it the distance I can run?

Is it how pretty I deem myself or society deems me?

Is it the amount of external validation I receive?

Is it whether or not I have a significant other?

Is it other people's opinion of me?

Is it how many followers I have or how many likes or comments I get on social media?

Is it how much I've accomplished?

Is it how productive I am on a given day?

Is it the amount of money I make?

It's easy to start basing our self-worth on these things. Really easy. I still find myself falling into these traps occasionally, and I have to consistently work to let it go over and over again. Because even though I forget sometimes, I know at my core that none of these things defines me.

We are inherently worthy because we exist.

It's not because of what we look like or what we do. Developing the ability to radically accept our bodies and recognize our value regardless of what we look like is paramount if we ever want to feel at home and at peace with ourselves. Even more, if we ever want the ability to take up space in our lives and recognize that our voices and our opinions matter—that we have the ability to create and effect real change in our lives and in the world—we have to recognize that our bodies are not a measure of our worth.

We are more than our bodies.

That being said, perhaps the goal should be to spend our precious time with those who see us for more than our bodies.

The common experience for both the individuals show-

cased in the trailer of *Revenge Body* was wanting the validation and love of the people in their lives, romantically and
platonically. We've probably all had this feeling before. I
know I have. But what I've come to realize over time is that
I'm only truly interested in sharing my energy with people
who see me for more than my body. I am not interested in
relationships—either romantic or platonic—in which I *ever*
have to consider if the size or shape of my body is going to
change the way someone feels about me. If a relationship is
going to cause me to question my worthiness or make me
feel like I need to manipulate my body in some way, it's not
a relationship I'm interested in maintaining. I'm not interested in earning anyone's love or affection.

That's not to say that people's thoughts about our bodies
or rejection of us won't hurt. They definitely have the potential to cause us emotional pain, but in those moments, I
try to remind myself that rejection is the universe's protection. If someone doesn't love, accept, and value me for who
I am, then they don't deserve me. After the initial frustration and some deep breathing and reflection, I also know
that other people's anti-fat bias is a reflection of them, not
me. I'm not the problem. Their internalized fatphobia is the
problem. The same is true for you as well.

As I previously stated, we simply cannot diet our way
into loving ourselves or into being accepted by others. After the pounds are shed and we are donning new clothes—
the ones we dreamed about wearing when we finally felt
like we looked good enough for them—we quickly realize

that the joy we thought we felt was fleeting, and we are still left with the same insecurities and worries and unhealed wounds. We just have a smaller body to reside in. And even more detrimental to our emotional well-being is the fact that the praise we receive because of our new body, which is likely coming from the people we were dying to have accept us, reinforces our worst fears. Thus it feels like the dominant cultural belief is in fact true—*our body is a measure of our worth*—and now we have the proof to back it up. The people closest to us *do* value us more when we are in a thin body.

It feels like a self-fulfilling prophecy, but in actuality we just haven't found the right people yet. The people that love us despite our bodies, not because of our bodies. What I want for myself and for every single person reading this is that we fill our lives with people and relationships that feed our soul. Relationships that allow us to fall more deeply in love with ourselves because we feel so nourished and cherished by our community that we never doubt who we are or how truly special we are, simply because we exist. May we all find our people—the people that treasure us because of who we are, not because of what we look like, and may we find the courage to let go of those individuals who don't see us that way.

What most people, myself included, find challenging is that it sometimes feels really difficult to remember that our bodies are not a measure of our worth when we are constantly inundated with messages that might lead us to believe that romantic love and even a sense of belonging would be easier to come by if we were in a smaller body. We repeatedly see people celebrated and praised for being in a smaller body, especially without any regard to the myriad of reasons it could be smaller, even if they're harmful reasons (e.g., chronic illness, grief, depression, eating disorders, etc.). The work is to remind ourselves that, ultimately, the love we truly desire is not dependent on the size of our bodies. Collectively dismantling diet culture and refusing to participate in its harmful systems by withholding our capital, both social and financial, allows us to begin to hold these systems accountable for the damage they have done (and continue to do) and the impact they've had on our relationships, while leading us on the path to collective liberation.

I recognize this is a tall order, and while we work toward this, I want to share a few tips with you to help you combat all the troubling messaging and feel at home and at peace with your body, because there will undoubtedly be days where you question your inherent worthiness, days when perhaps someone or something—maybe even someone you love, or thought you loved—begins to influence how you feel about your own body and its worthiness.

1. Show yourself compassion

Compassion is the antidote to feelings of guilt, shame, and dissatisfaction about our bodies. Some days we will love what we see and other days we won't—that's natural, and it's human. The trick is to learn to approach the feelings that come up, both good and bad, with curiosity and kindness and to always remember that regardless of how we feel about our bodies day to day, we are always worthy. We are often really good at having empathy and compassion for others—even for people who treat us like trash—but we sometimes (and by "we," I really mean "I") struggle to do that for ourselves. Like, why are we so damn hard on ourselves? Honestly, why?

I'm really hard on myself. A lot. Not about my body very often these days, but it definitely creeps up in other areas of my life—like writing this book for example. I go to therapy once a week because I have a lot of shit to work through. One week I was lamenting to my therapist about how I was experiencing some anxiety related to writing. "What if people think it's trash?" "What if no one buys it and my career is finished and I have to move back home and live in my mom's basement?" "Maybe this was just a bad idea . . ." After she let me go on for a while, my therapist stopped and asked me a question: "Is that you talking, or is that your inner bully?" Deep sigh. Of course it was my inner bully. So when my inner bully is working overtime and being particularly mean, I have to stop and remember to show myself a whole heap of love and compassion. And maybe this anecdote is helpful for you when you feel yourself struggling to treat yourself with kindness or to not be upset with your body. Is that you, or is that your bully? If it's your bully, maybe love on yourself a little harder.

2. Practice gratitude for yourself as a daily ritual

The way we look is the least interesting thing about us. Practicing gratitude for ourselves, independent of our physicality, helps us realize that we are so much more than our exterior. Our bodies are merely the shell we reside in and allow us to have this human experience. Show appreciation to yourself daily for things that have nothing to do with what you look like. If you ever find yourself struggling with this part, ask your best friend or someone who loves you deeply and unapologetically for some positive affirmation. I promise they will have a laundry list of amazing, awesome things they could say about you, and they would love to do that for you.

3. Stop comparing yourself with others

Comparison truly is the thief of joy, and comparing our perceived worst to other people's best can be downright harmful. We are our own worst critics, and social media makes it particularly easy to measure ourselves against others. When we are always viewing someone's highlight reel, it can sometimes make us feel down about our own lives. Here's a little reality check: No one's life is as good as it appears on social media. In case you have ever looked at my life on social media and thought it's all rainbows, travel, and sunshine, you are wrong. Here's a snapshot into my life at the moment I'm writing this. It's Friday evening (7:33 p.m., to be exact). I haven't left the house all day except to go to the bodega on the corner to get a Coke Zero and salt-and-vinegar chips (the dinner of champions), I've been wearing the same clothes since Monday (yes, I've showered but only to return to the same clothes), and the only things in my refrigerator are eggs and LaCroix. In other words, I'm a hot-ass mess right now. Don't let social media fool you, okay?

But I also encourage you to stop comparing the you of today with the you of the past. It's not about what your body used to look like or how it used to perform. It's about embracing the present. We can choose to love what is instead of comparing ourselves with what used to be. The you right now in this very moment deserves your love and adoration.

4. Cultivate a deep love affair with yourself

You are whole, complete, and unconditionally loved. Treat yourself with that regard. Celebrate and affirm yourself daily. We can beat ourselves up for all the things we are not, or we can choose to love ourselves with reckless abandon. Guilt and shame haven't worked so far, so why not give love a try?

You have to learn to be your own hype woman. I am blessed with a lot of friends who hype me up. They really do. Like, they think I'm dope as well, and I love and appreciate them for that. But also, I have to think I'm dope as hell. Every day I wake up and tell myself I'm a brilliant writer. The first time I did that, it was hard AF. It felt way too audacious to say. But if I don't believe that I'm a brilliant writer, who will? News flash: We gotta stop being so modest about how fly we are. It's gotta stop. Love yourself unabashedly. Hype yourself up. Sing your praises loudly. And I want you to feel it and mean it deep within your soul. There's enough sun for all of us to shine, my friends. We are all magic. The world needs to see all of us exhibit that.

I SHARED EARLIER IN THIS CHAPTER A STORY ABOUT A TERRIBLE man I dated. So naturally I have to end the chapter by telling you about how I went on to meet my Prince Charming, a man who loves me for exactly who I am. He is kind and caring and generous. He has looks that rival Michael B. Jordan's, and his personality is comparable to Russell Wilson's. He is everything that I could have ever imagined and more. That would be a phenomenal way to end this chapter. However, it's not true. Ya girl is still single AF. But having been single over the past couple of years, I've realized that falling in love with yourself is truly the greatest love story of all time. It's the best romance novel that could ever be written. The more deeply in love with yourself you fall, the less you can be convinced that your worthiness lies in your body.

In her book *All about Love*, bell hooks writes: "In an ideal world we would all learn in childhood to love ourselves. We would grow, being secure in our worth and value, spreading love wherever we went, letting our light shine. If we did not learn self-love in our youth, there is still hope. The light of love is always in us, no matter how cold the flame. It is always present, waiting for the spark to ignite, waiting for the heart to awaken and call us back to the first memory of being the life force inside a dark place waiting to be born—waiting to see the light."

In hindsight, I'm grateful for that text from my ex. It showed me the importance of knowing my own value and worth and not having it hinge on the opinion of someone else. While I do hope to be in a relationship again someday, I know what I want more than ever before. I know that when I find a love that feels so familiar, the kind of love that makes you feel so at home with yourself, I know it's because that person is just a reflection of me. That person won't be the magic. That person will simply illuminate the magic in me. I am already worthy. And so are you.

If you walk away from this chapter with nothing else, I hope you'll walk away knowing this:

You are worthy of love.

You are worthy of adoration.

You are worthy of joy.

You are worthy of respect.

You are worthy of happiness.

You are worthy of peace.

You are worthy of your dreams.

You are worthy of every good thing life has to offer you.

Right now, at this very moment. You are completely worthy.

It's not the size or shape of your body that determines that. You are inherently worthy because you exist.

From Principle to Practice

—

1. If you're completely honest with yourself, where are you deriving your worthiness from?

2. Is there a time when you have allowed your relationship status to affect your self-worth? Or have you stayed in a relationship with a partner who made you feel less than because you didn't feel worthy or deserving of more?

3. In what ways or areas of your life have you prohibited yourself from doing certain things due to the size of your body? Have you not worn certain items of clothing? Have you not gone on trips? Have you avoided taking pictures?

4. In what ways have you allowed your feelings about your body to cloud your accomplishments in life? Journal about a specific time when you allowed body obsession to cloud a life experience.

Our Liberation Must Be Collective:
Passing on Body Liberation to Others

WHILE I'VE LONG SINCE RELEASED THE NARRATIVE THAT I NEED to shrink my body, it took me longer to realize I was shrinking in other areas of my life. It took me longer to examine my own internalized anti-Blackness—how my own internalized white supremacy conditioned me to shrink my Blackness and cling to respectability politics, to fall back into the shadows.

I was shrinking my voice, suppressing everything that made me magical, and it was all rooted in fear. But here I am, standing in front of the world taking up space as a bold, beautiful, and magical Black woman.

At a certain point, I just decided that I was done focusing on shrinking—my body, my voice, my talents and abilities, my life. Standing at nearly six feet, I not only physically take up space, but I'm now fully invested in taking up space in all areas of my life. I used to worry about what people might think about me, as a Black woman, entering spaces where I didn't always feel welcome or celebrated. Now I realize that's not my burden to bear.

When we unlearn the scripts and release the social constructs we've been taught since birth, we free ourselves. The moment we unlearn something about ourselves is the moment we open ourselves up to learn who we really are—to meet the untamed versions of ourselves.

Most of us grew up with people telling us to "quiet down," "be less opinionated," "simmer down," "speak when spoken to," "be more ladylike," and countless other variations of ways to tell us that we shouldn't express ourselves too much. Along the way, we learned to be afraid to take up too much space in the world. These messages came from people who likely meant well and wanted to keep us safe, but they were misinformed. They themselves had been victims of the patriarchy, so they were only passing down the same lessons they had been taught. But those messages keep us small and keep us distracted.

I started blogging back in 2016, when I was working with a business coach, Jill Coleman. At the time, I was working with Jill to build an online fitness business, which, with her assistance, I did. When I first got into the fitness space as a coach and trainer, I played it safe for a long time. I blogged about things that I thought a trainer was supposed to blog about—workouts, tips for a healthy lifestyle, etc. In hindsight, it was bland and vanilla. It wasn't that those blogs weren't helpful or didn't contain useful information; it was that I wasn't being my authentic self. I was trying to fit in with mainstream fitness, a space that was super white, super thin, and super privileged. But in my private life, I was talking about racism, feminism, the patriarchy, and white supremacy, while reading the work of Audre Lorde, bell hooks, and James Baldwin. The reason I didn't merge these worlds is pretty simple. I was worried that I would be viewed as just an Angry Black Woman, a stereotype that depicts Black women as aggressive, overbearing, sharp-tongued, difficult, and bitter. So I played it safe for a long time. I wrote about the things I thought I *should* write about.

In 2017, I was really getting antsy and bored with the content I was creating. As a Black woman in the fitness space, I was growing increasingly frustrated with the lack of representation. That's what I called it then. In later years, I would just call it what it was—racism. I started writing this blog post on the topic and discussed it with Jill. She encouraged me to lean in and be my authentic self and talk about whatever was important to me. I still wasn't so sure that I was ready for that, so I sat on it for months. Literal months. Finally, in June 2017, Jill asked me what happened to that blog post I had been working on, and I admitted that I was actually a little nervous to release it. She basically told me to shit or get off the pot, reminding me in so many words that I could spend the rest of my life worried about not wanting to ruffle feathers or I could be a changemaker, but I couldn't be both.

A couple weeks after this conversation, I posted the blog, which was entitled "Is Fitness Only for Thin White Women?," on my website, ChrissyKing.com. It's important to note that at this time I had fewer than a thousand Instagram followers and no one—and I mean no one—was really reading my blog. Nonetheless, I was terrified. At the time I was still working my corporate job, so I intentionally posted the blog when I was traveling for work and had to be away from the internet for several hours. I call it the old "post and run." Roughly four hours later, I hesitantly opened my social media accounts to see what the verdict was. The unimaginable had occurred. People were reading the blog, and not only that, they were actually sharing it. It was resonating with folks. I had also received dozens of DMs and Facebook messages from people who told me they felt deeply seen and heard through my words, that I had captured the feelings they had been having for some time and expressed them for the world to understand.

Posting this blog felt like ripping off a Band-Aid. The anticipation was much worse than the actual event. I let go of the fear that had been holding me back and decided that the things I had been wanting to talk about were important and necessary, even though they weren't popular and trendy yet. More importantly, I realized that my feelings weren't my feelings alone. There were thousands of people who read that little blog. It gave me the courage to keep pushing the boundaries. To go deeper. To share all the things that had been bubbling in my heart. Not just because sharing my words is personally gratifying, but because I really believed that I could make a little difference in my corner of the internet—and maybe, someday, in the world.

> *When I dare to be powerful, to use my strength in the service of my vision, then it becomes less important whether or not I am unafraid.*
>
> —Audre Lorde

The sentiment of Audre's words has guided me from the moment I posted that first blog, and it continues to guide me every single day. I do most of the things I do afraid. I'm not immune to impostor syndrome. I wake up some days and wonder if I'm making enough of an impact. I have moments when I question who I am to dare to desire to change the landscape of the wellness industry. I have had all those thoughts many times over. But what I think of even more is how much body liberation changed me. How much it freed up my mental energy and well-being. It's because of body liberation that I have been able to change the trajectory of my life.

It's because of body liberation that I, a Black girl from Wisconsin, decided to leave my old life behind and move to Brooklyn. It's because of body liberation that two years after moving to NYC I got the chance to speak about body liberation in Times Square. It's because of body liberation that you're reading these pages. When I was a child, you could find me reading books and writing stories. I always thought I wanted to be a writer when I grew up, but by the time I got to college, I had decided to be more practical and major in something that would secure me a job. Writing was a memory long gone. My journey with dieting, strength training, and body image eventually led me back to the very thing I always wanted to do. I don't consider that an accident.

Body liberation set me free. When I found body liberation, I also liberated myself from thinking that I was never enough; I finally realized that not only was I enough, but I had always been more than enough. I finally realized that I had a very specific magic to share with the world, and it had nothing to do with what I looked like. And it's not only for my own benefit. I strongly believe that my ability to find body liberation is also the pathway to help others discover the same for themselves. Who knows how many people will be changed by the words I write, but ultimately, if one person finds their way to body liberation because of it, then it was all worth it.

That's true for each and every one of us. When we free ourselves from the confines of diet culture and body obsession, we open the floodgates for others to do the same. We seek liberation for ourselves, but ultimately, the goal is that we take that newfound energy—the energy that we had previously been spending obsessing about our bodies—

and we dismantle white supremacy and systems of oppression.

Imagine the change we could create in the world if we started breaking more molds. If we started standing in our power and didn't feel the need to shrink ourselves—physically, mentally, emotionally. If we truly embodied anti-racism, strengthened our ability to face our discomfort, and set about the work of ensuring that everyone, regardless of body size or identity, be treated with dignity and respect.

Here's the reality: We can spend our energy focusing on shrinking and obsessing about our bodies, or we can use our energy on creating magic and change in the world. We can leave our mark on the world or we can play small. It's really hard to do both. I would argue it's impossible. My life's work is not to shrink, and neither is yours. Now more than ever, the world needs us to show up powerfully and confidently. The days of sitting by the sidelines in silence are over. There's no magic in playing small.

Your greatest gift to the world is being your true self unapologetically. You're doing the world a disservice when you choose otherwise. Someone is waiting to see you shine. Someone is waiting to be inspired by you. Someone needs to see you free. Be confident. Be bold. Be assertive. Be whatever you want to be. That's when we begin to step into our power. That's when we can begin to take up space in our lives. For years, I've talked on my Instagram about the need to Take Up Space in the world, especially for women. There is power in deciding that you are done shrinking—your body, your talent, and your ambition—and deciding to take up space. I used to blindly give the advice that "there's no such thing as taking up too much space in the world." I still love the power phrase "Take Up Space" and still believe in its utility.

However, I also want to introduce some caveats. I was 100 percent wrong when I said there's no such thing as taking up too much space in the world, because there is. We take up too much space when we fail to realize that our voice may not be the one that needs to be heard right now; perhaps our issues aren't the ones that need to be elevated at the moment. For members of the dominant group, I can't stress this enough. It is 100 percent possible that you may be taking up too much space in certain arenas. It's entirely possible that there are folks who have more intersecting identities than your own who need the ability to take up more space, and sometimes that can happen only when you take up less space—when you realize that for far too long, people with your identity have been centered and it's time for that to change. We have to be able to recognize when individuals who look like us are taking up too much space at the table and have the foresight to take a step back and center others. This can feel challenging sometimes, because when you're accustomed to privilege, equality seems like oppression. But this is the work of actual liberation. It doesn't happen by mistake. It's intentional and requires something from us.

For all my white readers, I say this with all the love and compassion in the world, but Black people and other people of color need our own spaces sometimes. We need the ability to process and find community, absent the white gaze. So when we say that events or online communities are for BIPOC only, respect and honor that. It's not racist, and it doesn't mean we don't like white people. In a world where Black people feel the need to code-switch, flipping between standard English and African American Vernacular English almost daily, being among our own is our space to unmask and take off our armor, the armor we have to wear to protect ourselves in a white supremacist culture.

My sister, an avid yogi, was attending a virtual yoga session during 2020, shortly after the murder of George Floyd, that was specifically for Black women. It was advertised as such and explicitly stated this on the website before you could even register. It was meant to be a space of healing and communion from all the collective grief and trauma being experienced. On the day of the event, a white woman showed up, stating that she was "an ally and married to a Black man." This is an example of taking up too much space. This is white privilege. This is being more concerned about yourself than collective liberation. And while you may think this story sounds wild, situations like this occur way more often than you may realize. White people are often so used to being in and having access to everything that being excluded from a space feels like a personal attack.

But instead, they should support the liberation of everyone by respecting folks' boundaries.

I'm not saying to shrink your life. I'm saying to be more cognizant of when it's necessary to sit back and allow the voices of others to be heard more clearly. It's having the capacity to recognize when certain spaces aren't for you. I strongly dislike when people say they are a "voice for the voiceless." No one is voiceless; people just aren't listening to them because they're too busy holding the mic and being the expert. It's the same as when we speak of giving someone "a seat at the table." Giving someone a seat at the table still implies that the power and privilege are controlled by the person allowing others to join them. We can't achieve liberation for all of us when any one of us is trying to maintain power and privilege.

But in terms of the physical body, I think you should take up all the space. All of it. In a world that tells us that shrinking our bodies is the best thing we could do, I want you to take up as much space as you would like. We were not created to shrink. In the physical sense, there actually isn't such a thing as taking up too much space, except for maybe walking down the middle of the sidewalk without regard for others or not respecting people's personal space in the grocery store. Don't do that. That literally just makes you an asshole.

Our liberation truly is bound in each other, and when we keep that as our guiding principle, we can make decisions for our lives based not only on our own best interests but also on the best interests of the collective. I want us all to live our biggest and boldest lives, but I want us all to do it mindfully.

Systems do not maintain themselves; even our lack of intervention is an act of maintenance. Every structure in every society is upheld by the active and passive assistance of other human beings.

—Sonya Renee Taylor, author of
The Body Is Not an Apology

The goal of body liberation is that we all experience the joy of true liberation. Once we are moving toward that, the focus of our work has to move beyond just our individual ability to feel good in our own bodies. We must demand justice for all bodies, especially the most marginalized. However, if the base of our work in this space is not firmly rooted in anti-racism and dismantling diet culture and white supremacy, while continuously acknowledging our individual access to privilege, power, and opportunity, we fail to see that instead of dismantling the system, we are likely adding to it. Abolishing a system entails action on our part.

Without inner change, there can be no outer change. Without collective change, no change matters.

—angel Kyodo williams, writer and activist

White supremacy and the patriarchy affect us all—even if you are white. None of us are immune, although it affects some of us more than others. A white friend of mine and I were discussing this: how we are all affected by white supremacy on multiple levels. Neither of us knows a lot about biology, but she mentioned the interconnected nature of trees—about their root systems and how they essentially talk to one other about their needs for survival. If the root system of a neighboring tree is rotting, the other trees are also at risk. Vice versa, when a root system is strong and thriving, the trees surrounding it also thrive. She likened the trees to humanity. How even when we don't fully acknowledge it, we are interconnected. What affects our root systems affects the systems of all humanity. I read a few articles about it and came across the following words in a Medium article titled "What Trees Can Teach Us about Community and Connection":

> *Like humans, trees are interconnected even when that connection isn't visible to the naked eye, sharing in the wonders of the world, each searching for contentment, fulfillment, and a sense of peace. And because trees are an interconnected community, if one aspect of one tree is affected or damaged, the collective whole feels the disturbance.*

There is no liberation unless we are *all* free to exist in our bodies without fear of harm, danger, or systemic oppression.

There is no liberation without sacrifice. If we aren't willing to pass up opportunities, money, and even relationships to demand justice AND equity, including financial equity, for all bodies, we aren't doing the work of body liberation.

Back to the words of Audre Lorde, with my two preferred changes so that liberation is not bound by gender: "I am not free while any [person] is unfree, even when [their] shackles are very different from my own. And I am not free as long as one person of Color remains chained. Nor is any one of you." I never stop referring to these words, because these words remind me that freedom is not individual.

Our personal liberation is the pathway to our collective liberation.

I recently read some commentary online from someone I deeply admire voicing that they don't care about if people love their bodies or not, they care about dismantling diet culture. And while I don't care so much about if you love your body specifically, I do care if you love yourself, which we have already established is really not about your body at all.

I want to collectively dismantle systemic oppression that makes it difficult for all of us to thrive. The same oppression that negatively impacts people living in larger bodies (from healthcare to employment discrimination). The same oppression that leads millions of people into disordered eating and body dysmorphia. The same oppression that keeps millions of us, especially women, stuck because we are literally afraid of getting fat.

I also want you to love yourself in addition to dismantling. Because loving yourself deeply is a beautiful act of self-care, and every single one of us deserves to be the protagonist of our own love story. It is the greatest love story of all time. I will not ever downplay the gravity of loving yourself while living in a capitalist, white supremacist culture. It's undeniably difficult and some days will feel harder than others, but it's worth the fight. I will never wave the white flag in the face of white supremacy. It's already stolen so much from me—from us all. I may not live long enough to see the end of systemic body oppression, discrimination, and white supremacy, but I'll never stop working toward that. And while I work on that, I'm going to love on myself hard. Because that's what my ancestors would want for me, and I'm worthy of that. Joy is my birthright. Love is my birthright.

We have 50 percent of our population—millions of girls and women—devoting their brilliance and mental capacity and emotional intelligence to shrinking their waistlines instead of expanding their lives.

—Susan Hyatt, life coach

As I end this book, I'm asking you to join me in deciding that you are no longer going to be part of the 50 percent of the population giving the best of yourself—of your energy, of your magic, of your humanity—to the pursuit of being a smaller version of yourself. It's difficult, especially in the face of systemic oppression, to forgo chasing thinness, but it's one of the most loving acts we can do for ourselves. In fact, choosing your sanity and mental health over diet culture is not only an act of rebellion but an act of liberation. When you set yourself free, you give others the courage and inspiration to set themselves free as well.

I'm also asking you to join me in the pursuit of collective body liberation. Once we have experienced true body liberation for ourselves, we take that newfound joy and allow it to fuel our passion for everyone to experience that freedom. That is what fuels me daily. I don't pretend to have all the answers. I definitely won't pretend like I got everything right in this book. I'm far from perfect. But if I waited to get it perfect, I would have never written this book. I'm learning and growing and changing every single day, and I will be until I take my last breath. But body liberation has changed me in such a profound way that I can't imagine not sharing this message with the world in the hope that at least one more person will experience it as well.

The revolution needs you. You are magic. You are meant to do more with this life than to shrink yourself. Be bold. Be vibrant. Be unapologetic. Have the audacity to love yourself deeply. Release the social constructs. Rewrite your narrative. Show up. Free yourself and then work to free us all. You are a gift to this world.

Body liberation is a journey, and there is no five-step process to get there. I used to read every self-help book I could get my hands on because I desperately wanted someone to just tell me what to do, to tell me how to fix myself. But here's the thing: We aren't broken. We are humans navigating life and learning and growing as we do it. I can't possibly tell you the steps you need to take to achieve body liberation. It's a practice—one that never ends, if I'm being honest. It requires massive mindset shifts in a world that will daily attempt to convince you that it's not possible to achieve. You will have to fight for it. Diet culture and white supremacy will likely draw you back in over and over again, because we are literally immersed in it. It surrounds us on every side. It's the air we breathe. But as you embark on this journey, always lead with love, compassion, and grace for yourself.

Liberating our bodies, hearts, and minds from internalized oppression takes time, energy, and lots and lots of love. We need to believe we are worth the effort. And, we need to find others who are in for the journey too.

—Kate Johnson, *Radical Friendship*

My trip to Spain was a milestone for me because it was when I finally realized just how different my relationship with my own body had become. When I reflect, there wasn't one particular action that helped me get to liberation. It was each small loving act of kindness that I showed myself. It was all the difficult moments of sitting in the discomfort. It was doing the difficult work of addressing anti-Blackness and anti-fatness in my own life. It was deciding to stop caring about what everyone else thought about me and deciding to prioritize what I thought of me. It was processing grief and letting go of old versions of myself and body that didn't exist anymore. It was learning to embrace every part of myself for what I was—not what I wished I was.

For those of you still on the journey to liberation, you will have your own moment. One day you will simply notice just how much your relationship with your body has changed and, as a result, how much your life has changed, and when it happens, I hope you email me. Those are the kinds of emails I will gladly accept: the emails letting me know that you have tasted freedom, and you are now working to dismantle the systems, in your own way, because you understand how powerful body liberation is.

My hope is that you walk away feeling emboldened to embrace the body you have now, without condition, and the freedom to embrace it in all its iterations. And I hope that it changes us in such a profound way that we work to change the narrative so that those coming after us don't have to fight against the same harmful effects. So our sons and daughters might be born into a kinder, gentler society—one that nourishes liberation for all.

From Principle to Practice

———

1. How are you committed to working toward your own personal body liberation with compassion and kindness?

2. What personal sacrifices are you willing to make in the quest for collective liberation?

3. How are you committed to showing up differently for BIPOC and other members of traditionally excluded communities?

4. What comforts are you willing to part ways with?

5. What actions can you commit to, in this moment, to disavow and work to dismantle diet culture?

6. What actions are you going to take to ensure that you continue the work of anti-racism for the duration of your life?

7. When you witness friends, family members, coworkers, and peers engaging in fatphobia and harmful body narratives, how do you plan to respond?

8. In what ways are you willing to take on greater responsibility for the sake of collective liberation?

ACKNOWLEDGMENTS

Believe it or not, this was one of the most challenging parts of the book for me to write. I procrastinated as long as I possibly could. The manuscript was in its third round of edits before I finally hunkered down to write this. It's a lot of pressure. What if I forget to mention someone super important? What if I don't sound grateful enough? What if I do too much and come across like I'm writing a Grammy speech instead of the acknowledgment section of a book? Now can you understand why I've put this off?! So let me go ahead and relieve some of the pressure for myself. If I forgot to mention you and you know how helpful you have been to me, please charge it to my head and not my heart. I promise I appreciate you. In fact, you can feel free to call me and tell me that I forgot you and I will verbally apologize and make it right.

First of all, to my family, thank you for always supporting me. To my mom, it's clear that I thought I knew what I was doing from the moment I came out of the womb. I've always been determined to figure things out on my own and I'm positive I've given you more headaches than you care to admit. Thank you for never attempting to squelch my independence and for providing unending support, even when you haven't understood my decisions. To my sister, Celina, you are my ride or die. I would say that you are Solange in this situation, but that would make me Beyoncé and that doesn't seem fair. However, you do go hard for me, and you almost did fight someone in an elevator for me, so there are a lot of similarities when I really think about it. Even though you are my baby sister, you are the one always looking out for me, and I never have to question your loyalty. Thank you for being a cheerleader, a hype woman, and the best sister I could ever ask for. To my brothers, Chris and Corey, thank you for your support and honestly, where would I be without the nickname "Jolly Green Giant" that you so lovingly bestowed on me?

To my friends—Shirin Eskandani, Ashley Tucker, Allison Tenney, Amara Brown, Shana Spence, Ken Ward, David King, Bria Parrish, Monique Melton, Claire Gould, Chrissy Chard, Erika Charlestown, Molly Gailbraith, and Melissa McLeod, you are all near and dear to my heart. Thank you for being part of my community. I appreciate you all so much.

To all my other friends who never stopped cheering me on and checking in, thank you so much. The encouragement you provided and the belief you have in me means the world to me. To every single one of you who sent texts, shot me Venmos for caffeinated beverages, and showered me with compliments about how magical the book was going to be, you saw me through the rough days.

To my amazing book agent, Wendy Sherman, you are so appreciated. After Rebekah Borucki introduced us (thank you, Rebekah, for being willing to lend your connections), you jumped into action and guided me through the process. You encouraged me to turn down my first book offer and sent me back to the drawing board to write a proposal, and it was the best thing you could have possibly suggested. You believed in me from the start. Thank you for going on this journey with me.

Richelle Fredson, you started out as my book coach, helping me craft my book proposal, but then along the way, we became friends, and I am forever grateful for that. You helped me bring my vision for this book to life and cheered me on relentlessly. Book coach isn't an accurate description of the magical work you do with your clients.

To my editor, Jill. Thank you for allowing me to work at my own pace, keeping me accountable, and being there to support me in whatever ways I needed. Working with you on this book was so seamless. You allowed me to write the book that I wanted to write and helped me bring it to the best version it could be.

To Phoebe Robinson and the entire Tiny Reparations team, thank you for taking a chance on me and allowing me the opportunity to write my first book and with such an amazing publisher. I remember our first Zoom call to talk about the proposal and the queen herself—PHOEBE ROBINSON—popped on to surprise me. I would love to say that I played it super cool, but I had zero chill. I had a full-on fangirl moment. As soon as that call ended, I knew Tiny Reps is where I wanted my book to land. Not because I was starstruck (although I was), but because I felt the energy from everyone on the team and I knew it was the right place to publish my book. I can now say that I was 100 percent correct. It was a literal dream. Thank you for making it such a joy.

And lastly, I'm going to take a page out of Phoebe's book and thank my damn self. I'm so proud of myself for all the leaps of faith I took over the past four years to get me to this point—leaving my corporate job to do my own thing, moving to NYC, launching my own courses. They all prepared me for this moment. Writing a book is harder than I anticipated it would be. I definitely romanticized the process. I imagined it to be very sexy; you know, like Carrie Bradshaw from *SATC*. However, it was mostly me writing in sweatpants, rotating from my couch to my desk and then my local coffee shop. I doubted myself a lot of times, but I never quit. For that, I'm so proud of myself. I did the damn thing.

NOTES

INTRODUCTION

9 **body dysmorphia, defined:** "Body Dysmorphic Disorder," Mayo Clinic, https://www.mayoclinic.org/diseases -conditions/body-dysmorphic-disorder/symptoms-causes /syc-20353938.

13 **The clinicians were also less:** "People of Color and Eating Disorders," National Eating Disorders Association, https:// www.nationaleatingdisorders.org/people-color-and-eating -disorders.

14 **from Common Sense Media:** "Children, Teens, Media, and Body Image," infographic, Common Sense Media, 2015, https://www.commonsensemedia.org/children-teens-body -image-media-infographic.

14 **Furthermore, this "horrifying new research":** Julie Zeilinger, "Majority of 10-Year-Olds Have Gone on a Diet, According to Horrifying New Research," Mic, January 22, 2015, https:// www.mic.com/articles/108956/majority-of-10-year-olds-have -gone-on-a-diet-according-to-horrifying-new-research.

14 *Journal of Black Psychology*: Germine H. Awad et al., "Beauty and Body Image Concerns Among African American College Women," *Journal of Black Psychology* 41, no. 6 (December 2015), https://www.ncbi.nlm.nih.gov/pmc/articles /PMC4713035/#R5.

15 **"I am not free"**: Audre Lorde, "The Uses of Anger: Women Responding to Racism" (speech, June 1981), BlackPast, https://www.blackpast.org/african-american-history /speeches-african-american-history/1981-audre-lorde-uses -anger-women-responding-racism.

19 **"I write for those women"**: Joan Wylie Hall, ed., *Conversations with Audre Lorde* (Jackson: University Press of Mississippi, 2004), p. 90, https://www.google.com/books/edition /Conversations_with_Audre_Lorde/5WE-bAYX0LMC.

CHAPTER ONE: UNDERSTANDING THE BASIC CONCEPTS

25 **"If you can understand"**: Shirin Eskandani (@wholehearted coaching), "This platform is one where I speak about," Instagram, June 12, 2020, https://www.instagram .com/p/CBVXribJDqo.

30 **"stems from the fat acceptance movement"**: Marquisele Mercedes, "The Unbearable Whiteness and Fatphobia of 'Anti-Diet' Dietitians," Medium, September 16, 2020, https:// marquisele.medium.com/the-unbearable-whiteness-and -fatphobia-of-anti-diet-dietitians-f3d07fab717d.

31 **"Arguably, much like the feminist movement"**: Stephanie Yeboah, "Why Are Women of Colour Left Out of Body

Positivity?," *Elle*, September 15, 2017, https://www
.elle.com/uk/fashion/longform/a38300/women-of-colour
-left-out-of-body-positivity.

31 **"body positivity has been co-opted":** Lizzo (@lizzo),
"Please use the body positive movement," TikTok, April 4,
2021, https://www.tiktok.com/@lizzo/video/694885068129
3917446.

32 **"Mainstream body positivity misses the mark":** Chrissy King
(@iamchrissyking), "Loving yourself is really important,"
Instagram, October 25, 2021, https://www.instagram.com/p
/CVeYdUyvpiQ.

35 **"a term used to describe expressions of feminism":**
Wikipedia, s.v. "white feminism," accessed September 28,
2022, https://en.wikipedia.org/wiki/White_feminism.

37 **Jessie Mundell, an online exercise coach:** Jessie Mundell
(@jessiemundell), "I am not a 'body positive' fitness trainer,"
Instagram, July 12, 2021, https://www.instagram.com/p
/CRO1YuEjunJ.

40 **greater risk for body image issues:** Hannah M. Borowsky et
al., "Feminist Identity, Body Image, and Disordered Eating,"
Eating Disorders 24, no. 4 (July–September 2016),
https://www.ncbi.nlm.nih.gov/pmc/articles/PMC4999297/.

41 **"Body image," as defined:** "Body Image," National Eating
Disorders Association, https://www.nationaleatingdisorders
.org/body-image-0.

46 **with only fourteen states:** Aallyah Wright, "More States
Consider Bills to Prohibit Discrimination Against Black
Hair," *Stateline*, March 31, 2022, https://www.pewtrusts.org

/en/research-and-analysis/blogs/stateline/2022/03/31
/more-states-consider-bills-to-prohibit-discrimination
-against-black-hair.

49 **"a celebration of our deepest humanity":** Tina Strawn (@ tina_strawn_life), "Heard somebody was asking for me," Instagram, August 8, 2021, https://www.instagram.com/p/CSUFc2drcyx.

CHAPTER TWO: WHY BODY LIBERATION IS NEEDED

60 **"characteristics that were deemed integral":** Taylor Mooney, "The Racial Origins of Fat Stigma," CBS Reports, August 20, 2020, https://www.cbsnews.com/news/fat-shaming-race -weight-body-image-cbsn-originals/.

63 **The term "intersectionality":** Lexico, s.v. "Intersectionality," https://www.lexico.com/en/definition/intersectionality.

64 **landmark study found that:** Rebecca Hersher, "Obese Women Make Less Money, Work More Physically Demanding Jobs," *All Things Considered*, NPR, November 8, 2014, https://www .npr.org/2014/11/08/362552448/obese-women-make-less -money-work-more-physically-demanding-jobs.

65 **A review of studies published:** Kelly Coffey, "The Shocking Ways Large Women Are Mistreated by Health-Care Providers," *Self*, July 18, 2017, https://www.self.com/story /weight-bias-and-health-care.

65 **Many retailers don't sell larger sizes:** Gili Malinsky, "The 'Fat Tax' Is Real. Here Are 5 Examples That Prove It's More Expensive to Be Plus-Sized," *Business Insider*, June 7, 2019,

https://www.businessinsider.com/fat-tax-examples-clothing
-fashion-flying-bikes-furniture-coffin-2019-6.

65 **The consequences of weight stigma:** "Weight Stigma,"
National Eating Disorders Association, https://www
.nationaleatingdisorders.org/weight-stigma.

67 **in a 2021 British *Vogue* article:** Giles Hattersley, "Adele,
Reborn: The British Icon Gets Candid about Divorce, Body
Image, Romance & Her 'Self-Redemption' Record," British
Vogue, October 7, 2021, https://www.vogue.co.uk/arts-and
-lifestyle/article/adele-british-vogue-interview.

67 **"Thank you for the birthday love":** Adele (@adele), "Thank
you for the birthday love," Instagram, May 6, 2020, https://
www.instagram.com/p/B_1VGc5AsoZ.

69 **"My body's been objectified":** Abby Aguirre, "Adele on the
Other Side," *Vogue*, October 7, 2021, https://www.vogue.com
/article/adele-cover-november-2021.

70 **the most combined Grand Slam titles:** James Walker-Roberts,
"Tennis News—the Best 40 Stats, from Grand Slam Wins to
Records, to Celebrate Serena Williams's 40th Birthday,"
Eurosport.com, September 26, 2021, https://www.eurosport
.com/tennis/tennis-news-the-best-40-stats-from-grand
-slam-wins-to-records-to-celebrate-serena-willliams-s-40th
-b_sto8554494/story.shtml.

71 **Here are just a few of the tweets and comments:** Dr. David J.
Leonard "Serena Williams: 'Ain't I a Champion?,'"
NewBlackMan (in Exile), July 8, 2012, https://www
.newblackmaninexile.net/2012/07/serena-williams
-aint-i-champion.html.

72 **In a 2013 article for *Rolling Stone*:** Stephen Rodrick, "Serena Williams: The Great One," *Rolling Stone*, June 18, 2013, https://www.rollingstone.com/culture/culture-sports /serena-williams-the-great-one-88694.

CHAPTER THREE: DECOLONIZING OUR THOUGHTS ABOUT OUR BODIES

78 **Decolonizing our minds:** "What Does It Mean to Decolonize Your Mind," Organeyez, August 9, 2021.

79 **"No one ever talks about the moment":** Carolyn C. Denard, ed., *Toni Morrison: Conversations* (Jackson: University Press of Mississippi, 2008), p. 152, https://books.google.com/books ?id=eV9_8v4pTzsC.

80 **respectability politics:** Dictionary.com, s.v. "respectability politics," https://www.dictionary.com/browse/respectability -politics.

84 **"The average American encounters":** Amy Roeder, "Advertising's Toxic Effect on Eating and Body Image," Harvard T.H. Chan School of Public Health, March 18, 2015, https://www.hsph.harvard.edu/news/features/advertisings -toxic-effect-on-eating-and-body-image.

85 **Standards of beauty are used as weapons:** Ayesha Faines (@ayeshakfaines), "Is it cool to quote yourself?" Instagram, January 18, 2018, https://www.instagram.com/p/BeFX HEyn3EA.

92 **unconscious bias:** "Unconscious Bias Training," University of California, San Francisco, Office of Diversity and Outreach,

https://diversity.ucsf.edu/programs-resources/training
/unconscious-bias-training.

93 **the study found that:** Bradley S. Greenberg et al., "Portrayals
of Overweight and Obese Individuals on Commercial
Television," *American Journal of Public Health* 93, no. 8
(August 2003): 1342–48, https://www.ncbi.nlm.nih.gov/pmc
/articles/PMC1447967.

99 **"The era of the big booty":** Yomi Adegoke, "Why Does a Black
Butt Only Look Good in White Skin?," *The Guardian*,
September 23, 2014, https://www.theguardian.com
/commentisfree/2014/sep/23/why-black-bum-only-good
-white-skin-cultural-appropriation.

101 **"Fatphobia" is "defined as":** B. E. Robinson, J. G. Bacon, and
J. O'Reilly, "Fat Phobia: Measuring, Understanding, and
Changing Anti-fat Attitudes," *International Journal of Eating
Disorders* 14, no. 4 (December 1993): 467–80, https://pubmed
.ncbi.nlm.nih.gov/8293029.

101 **Here are a few more stats:** Endocrine Society, "Weight
Cycling Is Associated with a Higher Risk of Death, Study
Finds," *ScienceDaily*, November 29, 2018, https://www
.sciencedaily.com/releases/2018/11/181129153837.htm;
"Statistics on Dieting and Eating Disorders," Monte Nido
Mountain Nest, https://www.montenido.com/pdf
/montenido_statistics.pdf.

CHAPTER FOUR: BREAKING UP WITH DIET CULTURE AND EXAMINING YOUR PRIVILEGE

117 **The most disturbing part:** Rebecca Stamp, "Average Person Will Try 126 Fad Diets in Their Lifetime, Poll Claims," *Independent*, January 8, 2020, https://www.independent .co.uk/life-style/diet-weight-loss-food-unhealthy-eating -habits-a9274676.html.

CHAPTER FIVE: ACKNOWLEDGING THE HARM YOU MAY BE CAUSING OTHERS, PART 1

136 **Black trauma porn:** Tina Charisma, "Trauma Porn and the Commercialisation of Black Pain," *tmrw*, June 18, 2021, https://www.tmrwmagazine.com/features/opinion/trauma -porn-and-the-commercialisation-of-black-pain.

140 **why the fitness industry should stop using "savage":** Chrissy King, "Words That Don't Belong to Us: Why It's Time to Say Goodbye to Using the Word 'Savage,'" ChrissyKing.com, https://chrissyking.com/stopsayingsavage.

142 **performative allyship:** Wikipedia, s.v. "performative activism," https://en.wikipedia.org/wiki/Performative_activism.

142 **an ally is an individual:** "LGBTQ Terminology," LGBTQ+ Center, Wake Forest University, https://lgbtq.wfu.edu /resources/lgbtq-terminology.

144 **"involvement and collaboration":** "Diversity and Inclusion Definitions," Ferris State University, https://www.ferris.edu/ administration/president/DiversityOffice/Definitions.htm.

145 **True equity means:** Mathilde Roux, "5 Facts about Black Women in the Labor Force," US Department of Labor Blog,

August 3, 2021, https://blog.dol.gov/2021/08/03/5-facts-about
-black-women-in-the-labor-force.

147 **the racial pay gap:** "MSL Study Reveals Racial Pay Gap in
Influencer Marketing," MSLGroup.com, December 6, 2021,
https://mslgroup.com/whats-new-at-msl/msl-study-reveals
-racial-pay-gap-influencer-marketing.

148 **study from Creative Investment Research:** Janet Nguyen, "A
Year Later, How Are Corporations Doing on Promises They
Made to Fight for Racial Justice?," Marketplace, May 24, 2021,
https://www.marketplace.org/2021/05/24/a-year-later-how
-are-corporations-doing-on-promises-they-made-to-fight
-for-racial-justice.

CHAPTER SIX: ACKNOWLEDGING THE HARM YOU MAY BE CAUSING OTHERS, PART 2

153 **"caucacity" is a "slang term":** Dictionary.com, s.v. "caucacity,"
December 21, 2020, https://www.dictionary.com/e/slang
/caucacity.

154 **a term for this, "toxic fitness culture":** Ilya Parker, "What Is
Toxic Fitness Culture?," *Decolonizing Fitness* (blog), June 17,
2020, https://decolonizingfitness.com/blogs/decolonizing
-fitness/what-is-toxic-fitness-culture.

163 **In his 2016 TED Talk:** David R. Williams, "How Racism
Makes Us Sick," TEDEd, May 2, 2017, https://ed.ted.com
/lessons/oRaEODBk.

163 **Black women are two to three:** "Racial and Ethnic Disparities
Continue in Pregnancy-Related Deaths," press release,
Centers for Disease Control and Prevention, September 5,

2019, https://www.cdc.gov/media/releases/2019/p0905-racial-ethnic-disparities-pregnancy-deaths.html.

163 **COVID-19 deaths among Black Americans:** "Health Equity Considerations and Racial and Ethnic Minority Groups," Centers for Disease Control and Prevention, accessed January 25, 2022, https://stacks.cdc.gov/view/cdc/91049.

166 **the spiritual-bypassing crowd:** Robert Masters, "Spiritual Bypassing: Avoidance in Holy Drag," https://www.robertmasters.com/2013/04/29/spiritual-bypassing; Zawn Villines, "What to Know about Toxic Positivity," *Medical News Today*, March 30, 2021, https://www.medicalnewstoday.com/articles/toxic-positivity.

166 **"The easiest way for white women":** Rachel Cargle (@rachel.cargle), "I don't want your love and light if it doesn't come with solidarity and action," Instagram, November 3, 2018, https://www.instagram.com/p/BpvQ6nnHh4o.

168 **"'You're soooo authentic,' I hear daily":** Kendra Austin (@kendramorous), "In case y'all forgot, you can catch me on my newsletter Come Home," Instagram, September 27, 2021, https://www.instagram.com/p/CUVNUuUguZY.

CHAPTER SEVEN: EMBRACING PLEASURE AND REVOLUTIONIZING OUR RELATIONSHIP WITH OURSELVES

177 **"It is no easy task to be self-loving":** bell hooks, *All about Love* (New York: William Morrow, 2001), p. 54.

197 **poet Upile Chisala:** Upile Chisala, "Nectar," in *a fire like you* (Kansas City, MO: Andrews McMeel Publishing, 2020),

https://www.google.com/books/edition/a_fire_like_you
/BnvNDwAAQBAJ.

CHAPTER EIGHT: GRIEF, REMORSE, AND THE MOURNING OF OUR BODIES

202 **"You can grieve the ending":** Alex Elle (@alex__elle), "Gentle Reminder: You can grieve the ending of something and also be grateful that it's over," Twitter, December 13, 2021, https:// twitter.com/alex__elle/status/1470550222698913796.

213 **entitled** *The Joy of Movement*: Kelly McGonigal, *The Joy of Movement: How Exercise Helps Us Find Happiness, Hope, Connection, and Courage* (New York: Avery, 2021), p. 3, https:// www.google.com/books/edition/The_Joy_of_Movement /WjsZEAAAQBAJ.

CHAPTER NINE: BOUNDARIES AND THE BODY

239 **some amazing ways to respond:** Nedra Glover Tawwab (@nedratawwab), "You can change your boundaries as needed," Instagram, October 11, 2021, https://www .instagram.com/p/CU5Cbp2A2rp.

CONCLUSION

282 **"What Trees Can Teach Us":** Aurora Eliam, "What Trees Can Teach Us about Community and Connection," Medium, January 22, 2021, https://medium.com/stories-by-aurora-e /what-trees-can-teach-us-about-community-and -connection-4987c8296517.

ABOUT THE AUTHOR

Chrissy King is a writer, speaker, educator, and former strength coach with a passion for creating a diverse and inclusive wellness industry. She empowers individuals to stop shrinking, start taking up space, and use their energy to create their specific magic in the world. With degrees in social justice and sociology from Marquette University, Chrissy merges her passion for social justice with her passion for fitness to inspire members of the wellness industry to create spaces that allow individuals from all backgrounds to feel seen, welcomed, affirmed, and celebrated.

chrissyking.com
🐦 📷 IAmChrissyKing